A WALK ALONG THE RIVER II

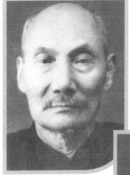

CHEN
DING-SAN

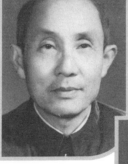

JIANG
ER-XUN

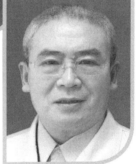

YU GUO-JUN

A WALK ALONG THE RIVER II

Transmitting a Medical Lineage
through Case Records
and Discussions

Yu Guo-Jun

TRANSLATED BY

Dan Bensky / Andrew Ellis / Craig Mitchell / Michael FitzGerald

EASTLAND PRESS ▶ SEATTLE

Originally published in 2006 by China Press
of Traditional Chinese Medicine as part of a larger
work entitled *Zhongyi shicheng shilu* (中医师承实录).
This English translation is authorized by the publisher.

English language edition © 2019 by China Press of Traditional Chinese Medicine,
Dan Bensky, Andrew Ellis, Craig Mitchell, and Michael FitzGerald

Cover photo © Jun Wei Fan

Published by Eastland Press, Inc.
P.O. Box 99749 Seattle, WA 98139, USA
www.eastlandpress.com

ISBN: 978-0-939616-89-3
Library of Congress Control Number: 2018968589

Printed in the United States of America
2   4   6   8   10   9   7   5   3   1

Cover design by Gary Niemeier and Patricia O'Connor
Book design by Gary Niemeier

Table of Contents

Translators' Foreword

The publication of the first volume of *A Walk Along the River* brought seven chapters of Dr. Yu's Chinese text to the English-reading public. This second volume picks up where the first left off and presents the remaining chapters. The translational approach that we applied to the first volume is continued here, so we refer the reader to the Translators' Foreword in the first volume for details. In short, our approach to the translation of this text is to present to the Western practitioner of Chinese medicine a translation that reads smoothly and yet does not sacrifice accuracy nor avoid or oversimplify the complexities of theory and practice.

As with the first volume, we have taken some liberties with the original text, usually in consultation with Dr. Yu, to increase readability and insure that the presented material is properly understood by the Western practitioner of Chinese medicine. Examples of these changes span from the simple removal of common nonsubstantive phrases to the addition of material that makes the presented material more accessible to the Western reader. An example of the former is the removal of the omnipresent phrase, "as everybody knows (大家都知道 *dà jiā dōu zhī dào*)." In Chinese, the phrase is common in everyday speech and gives no pause to the Chinese reader. In English, it seems completely unnecessary and is the first phrase our eighth-grade English teacher would remove.

Quite opposite to removing unneeded wording, we also added information that the English reader might need where the Chinese reader would not. In its simplest form the additions were rudimentary, as in changing the entry of 二地黄 *èr dì huáng* (literally 'two earth yellows') to Rehmanniae Radix *(shēng dì huáng)* and Rehmanniae Radix praeparata *(shú dì huáng)*. For more complex issues we often contacted Dr. Yu for clarification and incorporated his response directly into the text or into a question and answer in the case's discussion section. This type of translators' edit is seen in the chapter of the text on pediatric fever. Whereas the Chinese text simply states that the parents were advised to pay attention to the child's diet, we asked Dr. Yu what specific instructions were imparted to the parents, and in the English translation, added his response to the body of the text.

The minor liberties we have taken in our translation of the original text have been approved, and even encouraged, by Dr. Yu. As translators and practitioners of Chinese medicine, we have the utmost respect for Dr. Yu and want to point out that it is his accommodating attitude and meticulous attention to our constant questions that we hope have made this book and its first volume uniquely useful to English-language Chinese medicine practitioners.

Introduction

How I Came to Walk the Path of Chinese Medicine

From childhood I had a love of studying. In high school I was at the top of my class. In those days my achievements came more in the realm of the sciences, however I also enjoyed the humanities and social sciences. This prompted my teachers to say that I would "break the mold" and do something unprecedented in our community.

Because of the undivided attention that I gave to my studies, I became somewhat aloof from politics and everyday issues. That I was solely focused on non-political academic matters was noted by the school authorities and considered heterodox.

For example, I had one teacher who I thought lectured very well. I naively suggested that he consider writing a book in order to spread his teaching experience. Although I had no ulterior motive, he listened and hatched a plan. This sanctimonious teacher embellished the story and went behind my back to lodge a complaint with the authorities. He claimed that I was encouraging him to "set himself up as an authority."

What was even worse was then at a mass rally, the school leader, wearing a livid expression, and through gnashed teeth, scolded me for being "too big for my britches" and for being a "rabble rouser." The worst part of this event was that in the end, my graduation certificate was marked "emphasized academic knowledge over politics." This was a political black mark that could lead to devastating consequences. As a child I had already developed a strong desire to aid my own country and to alleviate suffering. The important works of Marxism, especially *Selected Works of Mao Zedong*, were among my favorite extracurricular reading. It was just that I did not know the ways of the world and so did not fall into the conventions of the time.

I persisted in my intention to participate in the 1964 university entrance examination. My first choice was the Beijing University philosophy department. My second choice was the political economics department at Sichuan University. Although my scores on the entrance examination far exceeded the cutoff for admission to Beijing University, I received no offers for admission from there or any other well-known school. In fact, even the admittance letter from Sichuan University took its time coming and was late.

After getting into school I found out that I had failed some parts of the test. Originally, the Sichuan University Provost, Liu Hong-Kang, who was a famous philosopher, economist, and linguist, did not admit me. However, while on his way to the school one day he passed the site in Chengdu where the famous Tang-dynasty poet Du Fu had a cottage. Something caused him to change his mind and he firmly decided to admit me to the political economics department. During my time at the university, I frequently visited the site of the cottage to remember this moment and to offer my sincere thanks to the spirit of the sage-poet, Du Fu.

My Path of Self Study

I began my own study of Chinese medicine purely by accident. It is a long story and one of the lucky coincidences of my life. It came about through a series of mishaps that led to a famous doctor rescuing me from dire straits.

In 1966 as a result of the Cultural Revolution, all classes at the university stopped. Some of my classmates and I were sent by the Sichuan Provincial Cultural Revolution Reception Center to investigate Dayi County and set up a Reception Station there. One day, when it was my turn on duty at the center, two country doctors came in to lodge a complaint. They reported that their teacher, Jian Yu-Guang, had been accused of "feudalistic superstition" by the Red Guards as a result of his use of "special pills" to treat patients. These special pills had been confiscated, his medical qualification was revoked, and seven of his students were implicated in the criminal investigation. They told me that Dr. Jian's pills were made from combinations of Chinese medicinal substances and that he had cured many people with conditions such as liver cirrhosis, cavitary tuberculosis, and severe uterine prolapse. I was amazed but also skeptical.

The next day I rode my dilapidated bicycle more than ten kilometers outside the city to the rural area where Dr. Jian practiced, called the Yuanxing Commune. I interviewed more than ten patients and determined that the reports were accurate. That same night I stayed up to write a report of my findings, and the next day I handed the report directly to the head of the county Party committee. With a sense of righteousness, I requested the "liberation" of Dr. Jian and his students. The committee head sought out the chief of the county public health branch to determine how to proceed with this situation. At that time, the words of the Red Guards had the force of an imperial edict, so it was a delicate situation.

Nevertheless, I was brimming with an insatiable curiosity about Dr. Jian's special pills and felt that I needed to quickly find a way to see these amazing effects with my own eyes. I applied to the county administrator to allocate funds for scientific research to support the work of Dr. Jian and his disciples in producing these special pills.

My high-minded rationale was that to provide support for this novel product would be, in the words of Chairman Mao, to "support new things to serve the health of the people." The county Party committee head agreed with my proposal and immediately ordered that the physics laboratory of the Dayi County middle school be used to conduct scientific inquiries into the special pills.

THE LEGEND OF THE FIVE-COLOR SALT ESSENCE

Dr. Jian's pills were called Five-Color Salt Essence. Aside from table salt, they also included native lake salt and Sulfur *(liú huáng)*. I watched the process of making the pills and was concerned about possible toxicity. After finishing the pills, Dr. Jian and I made a special trip to the Sichuan Provincial Research Institute, located in Huangjiaoya in Chongqing city, to request an evaluation of the pills. Thankfully, the evaluation revealed no toxicity and so I was able to set aside my concerns.

I decided to act quickly and petitioned the county head to provide money to establish the Dayi County Specialty Hospital for the treatment of chronic, intractable diseases. Dr. Jian oversaw the operation and we used his special pills in conjunction with Chinese herbal medicine. The treatment effects at the new hospital were remarkable and word spread far and wide. Our patient numbers increased exponentially. However, the hospital did not charge patients for care and the county budget was limited, so at a certain point it became difficult for us to continue.

Because of my concern about the future of the hospital, I wrote to the heads of the county public health bureau, the Chengdu College of Traditional Chinese Medicine, and the Chengdu Military Authority to seek support. Although Wenjiang Prefecture made the decision to establish the "Five-Color Salt Essence Research Group" with Dr. Jian and his disciples, I was still frustrated by the paucity of funds, the narrowness of the scope of research, and the slowness of the pace. Therefore, I continued writing letters and sharing materials with my superiors. One of my letters deeply moved the head of the Chengdu Military Authority and he sent out a directive, which caused the Military Authority and the Chengdu College of Traditional Chinese Medicine to deploy an investigator. Ultimately, the Research Group became a people's collective, led by Dr. Jian, called the Wenjiang Regional Chinese Herbal Research Institute. It was also known as the Chengdu City Research Institute.

MY FIRM RESOLUTION TO STUDY MEDICINE

Spurred on by my intellectual curiosity, I continued my work. Dr. Jian and his disciples told me that prior to meeting me, they had unsuccessfully sought out assistance on many occasions. They had petitioned for someone to oversee their research, but nobody was willing to help. However, after meeting me, it was as if "the clouds had been parted so that the sun could shine." Not only did I manage the situation, I saw it through to its completion. Was I not destined to study Chinese medicine?

I recalled Dr. Jian quoting the renowned Song statesman, Fan Zhongyan: "If you cannot be a wise minister, be a wise physician." This brought to mind Marx's schoolboy essay entitled, "Reflections of a Youth on Choosing a Profession." Marx believed that young people should select the profession that had the most potential to promote the well-being of the most people and that they should reject selfish considerations. I suddenly realized that given my uncertain future in the profession of political economics, I should become a physician. Because medicine was not classist, but was for the benefit of all human beings, this was even better than "the most people!"

However, as the Cultural Revolution was rolling along in full force, everyone was swept up in it and forced to go along. I strongly desired to escape that world, but it was easier said than done. I even looked over the 36 stratagems in *The Art of War* by Sun-zi, but none of them seemed applicable. However, I suddenly came up with a plan. I decided to fake an illness and was sent to the hospital ward within the school. I then went to the school library openly and borrowed many books about medicine. I closed the doors to my room and began to study, day and night. I was determined to follow the course that I had laid out for myself and I persisted through all obstacles.

It took me more than a year to work my way through the main textbooks of Western medicine and all of the current textbooks of Chinese medicine. After this time, I began to see patients, namely, my fellow students and teachers. When I say that I was "seeing patients," what I mean is that I was listening to their complaints, taking the pulse, looking at the tongue, and then going back to my books. I was just following the prescribed methods, but unexpectedly, I was getting results. One of the school doctors exclaimed that "through the study of books, Yu Guo-Jun will become famous!"

How to "learn clinically"

Outside the school gates there was an older doctor with excellent skills who worked in the communal clinic. Because he had been labeled a "counter-revolutionary," I could not go to him openly but would secretly go to see him in the evenings for his advice and guidance. He also loaned me some older thread-bound medical books to read.

The Provincial Public Hospital was only five kilometers from my school. Because the patient registration fee was very inexpensive, I would frequently go there and pretend to be a patient in order to observe the doctors. At that time, the clinic rooms were housed in simple, one-story buildings. I was able to stand outside the window or even sit on the windowsill and closely observe the process. Because the doctors had more patients than they could handle, they were too busy to ever worry about my "stealing their skills." In 2001, when I was answering questions related to a promotion to become a senior physician, I realized that one of the examiners was a physician I had "stolen from" during that time. When I laughed about it and told him this story, he was at first taken aback, but then joined in my laughter.

The Guiding Light of Zhang Xi-Chun

Zhang Xi-Chun shows the way

After finishing my self-directed study of Chinese medicine textbooks, I browsed many other books on Chinese medicine. Early one morning, while looking through the books in Dr. Jian's library, I happened upon the third volume of *Essays on Medicine Esteeming the Chinese and Respecting the Western (Yī xúe zhōng zhōng cān xī lù)*. Leafing through the book, a passage explaining Gypsum fibrosum *(shí gāo)* leapt out at me and I was immediately drawn into the text. Words failed me, and with a laser-focus on the text I read the entire passage immediately. I felt as if I had been enlightened! I sighed in wonder at the existence of such marvelous books about medicine. I read day and night, finishing not just the third volume, but also the first two volumes. I read each volume three times, taking extensive notes.

During that period of time I was drunk on the words of Zhang Xi-Chun and my mind was filled with his texts. All I talked about was Zhang Xi-Chun and sometimes I even dreamed that I was reading his books. I even boasted to my classmates that I had passed through a window of time and space to enter the thoughts of Zhang Xi-Chun.

Having studied the pithy prose of this exemplary physician, I didn't run into many roadblocks when I turned to other books on Chinese medicine, including the ancient, archaic, and profound texts of the Four Great Medical Classics: *Yellow Emperor's Inner Classic (Huáng Dì nèi jīng)*, *Discussion of Cold Damage (Shāng hán lùn)*, *Divine Husbandman's Classic of the Materia Medica (Shén Nóng běn cǎo jīng)*, and the *Classic of Difficulties (Nàn jīng)*. In the many years since, not a few new students have asked me how best to study Chinese medicine. I tell them that they should completely master one school of thought, be very familiar with a few schools, and have a basic understanding of many schools.

WITH GOOD FORTUNE I'M ABLE TO PROPERLY HANG OUT MY SHINGLE

From 1969-71, I worked on a military reclamation farm, doing physical labor and seeing the farmers as patients. Whenever I encountered a difficult disease, I would recollect passages from Zhang Xi-Chun. In those days, I was uneasy about picking up a book and consulting it while the patient was present, but right after they left, I would quickly look up their situation in the text. In the evenings, I continued my studies by the light of my kerosene lamp, deep into the night. During this time on the farm, I studied the *Discussion of Cold Damage (Shāng hán lùn)* and *Essentials from the Golden Cabinet (Jīn guì yào lüè)*.

In the fall of 1971, I was assigned to the Leshan special district where I just happened to meet a physician who was working in the Huatou Mountain region of Jiajiang County. He was a recent graduate of the Chengdu College of Traditional Chinese Medicine who had requested this assignment. After speaking with him, I decided to petition the county head to see if I could change my occupation and put myself forward as a Chinese medicine physician. One of the party secretaries said to me, "Given that your specialty is political economics, do you really know how to see patients?" One of the army officials chimed in, "Let him try. After a month, when it is clear that he is not succeeding, he can be reassigned." With great excitement, I hurried off to the Huatou area, 47 kilometers away, in a region of Jiajiang that was considered to be a challenging place to live due to the harsh conditions. The next day, I entered the Chinese medicine clinic of the Huatou Hospital and began my formal career as a physician. I began to apply the wide-ranging knowledge of difficult conditions that I had gleaned from the works of Zhang Xi-Chun and I rapidly gained experience in using his formulas.

For example, I encountered a woman who was about 50 with varicose veins in both her legs, which caused her so much pain that she limped into the clinic. The moment after she sat down, she began to cry. Apparently, she had been to several large hospitals and nobody would write a prescription for her. Never having treated this disease before, I just looked at the symptoms, which were clearly the result of blood stasis, and prescribed Zhang Xi-Chun's formula Fantastically Effective Pill to Invigorate the Collaterals *(huó luò xiào líng dān)* to which I added a large dosage of fierce medicinal substances to dispel blood stasis. After six packets, the patient's pain had greatly diminished. After more than 30 packets, the pain had resolved and her gait was essentially normal.

I used a variety of Zhang's formulas with excellent results for a range of complaints. I treated a post-stroke patient with hemiplegia using a modification of Sedate the Liver and Extinguish Wind Decoction *(zhèn gān xī fēng tāng)*, which rapidly brought the patient out of danger. I cured a patient of recalcitrant low back pain with Stimulate the Center Decoction *(zhèn zhōng tāng)*.[1] I used Harmonizing and Regulating Decoction *(xiè lǐ tāng)*[2] with the addition of Bruceae Fructus *(yā dǎn zǐ)* to cure a case of hot dysentery with tenesmus. Using Yin-Enriching Dryness-Clearing Decoction *(zī yīn qīng zào tāng)*,[3] I rescued a child from long-term diarrhea damaging the Spleen yin. I also effectively used a formula recommended by Zhang Xi-Chun, called Modified Tangkuei Decoction to Tonify the Blood *(jiā jiǎn dāng guī bǔ xuè tāng)*, to treat a woman with severe uterine bleeding.

A month after "hanging out my shingle," as expected, the county sent out a representative to evaluate my performance. The conclusion of the investigator was "satisfactory, contrary to expectations." These extremely simple and unadorned words of praise reminded me of the famous quote from Louis Pasteur, "Fortune favors the prepared mind."

Baby Steps

FREQUENTLY PUBLISHING ARTICLES

In the fall of 1973, after just two years beginning to formally practice medicine, I began to publish articles. At that time, I was only aware of one publication, entitled *New Chinese Medicine (Xīn zhōng yī)*. I submitted two articles and was fortunate to have both of them quickly published. When too much undeserved good fortune comes, it becomes difficult to continue doing things the same way. As my clinical experience was quite limited, I began to feel like an impostor. Chinese medicine is a science that emphasizes practical experience and I lacked training in the basic clinical skills. Not only did I feel like an impostor because of my limited clinical training, but also I had read so little and owned so few books. The more I relied on book knowledge, the more I realized with regret how much more I needed to read.

....

1. Stimulate the Center Decoction *(zhèn zhōng tāng)*: Atractylodis macrocephalae Rhizoma *(bái zhú)*, Angelicae sinensis Radix *(dāng guī)*, Citri reticulatae Pericarpium *(chén pí)*, Magnoliae officinalis Cortex *(hòu pò)*, Olibanum *(rǔ xiāng)*, Myrrha *(mò yào)*.

2. Harmonizing Decoction *(xiè lǐ tāng)*: Dioscoreae Rhizoma *(shān yào)*, Lonicerae Flos *(jīn yín huā)*, Paeoniae Radix alba *(bái sháo)*, Arctii Fructus *(niú bàng zǐ)*, Glycyrrhizae Radix *(gān cǎo)*, Coptidis Rhizoma *(huáng lián)*, Cinnamomi Cortex *(ròu guì)*.

3. Yin-Enriching Dryness-Clearing Decoction *(zī yīn qīng zào tāng)*: Talcum *(huá shí)*, Glycyrrhizae Radix *(gān cǎo)*, Paeoniae Radix alba *(bái sháo)*, Dioscoreae Rhizoma *(shān yào)*.

I suddenly thought that perhaps I had really gotten ahead of myself and was putting myself into the public eye prematurely. Once I realized this, I regretted putting myself out through these articles as though I was a knowledgeable physician. From that point on, I stopped writing and submerged myself in seeing patients by day and studying by night. I researched and read widely, selecting what I found valuable. I also benefited from the influence and stimulation of studying with the classical formula master, Dr. Jiang Er-Xun.

Five years later, I again set pen to paper and found that not only was my brain full of ideas, but expressing them on paper came naturally. During that period, I published in more than 20 different Chinese medicine journals. It should be noted that at that time authors did not pay for their manuscripts to be reviewed, nor did they pay for space on a page; selections were made based purely on the quality of the writing. I remember in 1981, following the publication of an article in the *Journal of Chinese Medicine (Zhōng yī zá zhì)* entitled "A Discussion of Zhang Xi-Chun's Treatment of the Spleen and Stomach," that I received a great deal of heartfelt encouragement. I then submitted several other manuscripts only to have them rejected. Because I placed at least some value on my writing, I took it upon myself to inquire why my articles had been rejected.

I received in response a beautiful hand-written letter explaining that the rate of acceptance for publication was only 3-5% of all submissions. Thus, when a manuscript was rejected, it was not necessarily of low quality, but rather that there was a very strict process that involved multiple reviews by different people prior to publication. It occurred to me that this must be why the *Journal of Chinese Medicine (zhōng yī zá zhì)* never seemed to publish anything that was substandard.

I began to reflect on why I, a low-level primary care physician, desired to write academic articles. Was I seeking fame and fortune? The Tang-dynasty poet Xu Yu wrote in *Feelings of Spring (Gǎn chūn)*, "Fame and fortune cannot stop one from aging, yet poetry and verse can rescue one from inadequacies." What was I seeking? Confucius wrote that, "Study without reflection leads to deception and thought without study leads to defeat." I took this to mean that studying texts without reflecting on them would lead one to be confused and that by merely pondering questions without studying the texts, one would become sloppy. Although Confucius does not specifically mention writing articles, it must be remembered that he represents an older time when he could simply state ideas that his students would organize and record. If his own students had followed the same oral tradition and written nothing down, we would not have the highly regarded *Analects (Lún yǔ)*! So, when I was young, I added my own doggerel postscript to the previous adage, "To think and study without writing leads to regret."

This notion of regret has two different aspects. First, our ancestors described three 'imperishables': attaining virtue, having meritorious achievements, and expounding on one's thoughts in writing. Writing an article connects one to posterity. Regardless of life's destiny, is it not a regret to not leave behind at least a few words and thoughts? Second, when we read a text, we are entering the thought process of another person. It is only when we write down our own ideas that we begin to follow the path of our own thoughts. Without writing down one's thoughts and ideas it can be difficult to fully think things out or to fully comprehend the pearls contained in someone else's writing.

My Meteoric Rise

In the fall of 1983, the famous physician Lu Gan-Fu of the Sichuan Provincial Chinese Medicine Research Institute, along with some of the leadership of that institution, out of the blue showed up at the rural hospital where I worked. He chatted with me for a couple hours, covering a wide range of topics. Not long afterward, I received a letter from Dr. Lu enthusiastically inviting me to come work with him at the Institute in Chengdu. I learned that Dr. Lu had received a recommendation about me from Jin Jia-Jun, the chief editor of *Sichuan Chinese Medicine (Sìchuān zhōng yī)*, whom I had never met. By year's end, I had transferred to the Institute's department on medical literature research. To those around me, this was considered a meteoric rise.

While at the Research Institute, I saw patients, studied, and wrote articles. While I felt more than up to the tasks I had to perform, I soon began to feel homesick. I was, after all, just a simple man from Leshan. Life in the big city, full of activity and noise, grew wearisome for me. My writing lacked inspiration and my hair began to turn grey.

Many times I began the process of seeking a transfer. However, to do this in a tactful way seemed impossible and the right words eluded me. I could not find a good excuse. It was extremely awkward. My difficulties evaporated when I discovered that there were plans to start an office in Leshan specifically for advanced students of Jiang Er-Xun and that I was being asked to assist. Only after Dr. Jiang himself came to Chengdu three times to discuss the new plans did I have a perfect and acceptable reason to leave.

Thinking back to a year earlier, when I had left my position in the countryside to move to Chengdu, I remembered that many of my colleagues from the hospital had turned out to wish me well. As I passed through Meishan, the hometown of Su Dong-Po, the words that the Tang poet Li Bai wrote upon his accepting an imperial edict to move to the capital suddenly came into my head: "I tilted my head up and laughed as I left home. For after all, am I not just a wild weed?" Truly, I had naiveté to spare, I was insufficiently mature, and I had carried with me my rustic manners.

When it came time to return, I ended up seated in the same vehicle that I had taken to Chengdu the year before. As the first faint rays of sun came into the car, I left Chengdu quietly without a single person there to see me off. I did not feel lonely, I just felt badly for perhaps not fulfilling the expectations of my benefactors in Chengdu.

During my time at the Provincial Research Institute in Chengdu, I had collaborated with a colleague, Huang Ming-An, on a reference text entitled *Collected Explanations of the Inner Classic and Classic of Difficulties (Nèi nàn jīng huì shì)*, which had been published by the Sichuan Science and Technology Press. In the Sichuan television station's introduction to our school's achievements in the field of scholarship on the ancient texts of Chinese medicine, they specifically recommended this book, lavishing it with extensive praise by saying such things as our volume should be considered the beginning of a new phase of research into these classical texts.

The Path of a Disciple

Being a disciple of the modern master of classical formulas, Jiang Er-Xun, did not occur because I was assigned to him, nor did we ever have a written agreement or any contract.

The relationship evolved out of my voluntary desire to work with him. It just happened naturally by itself and ended up being something that led to us all being satisfied.

Carrying on the work of organizing Dr. Jiang's clinical experience

When I began my professional career in medicine, Dr. Jiang was already a household name in Leshan. His fame and prestige did not come through advertising or through media reports. It arose gradually over many decades from successfully treating patients, and it was disseminated organically throughout the region. Dr. Jiang himself was the disciple of a legendary Sichuan physician, Chen Ding-San. Dr. Chen had read extensively, researched medicine deeply, and had an amazing memory. According to Dr. Jiang, Dr. Chen could not only recite from memory the *Discussion of Cold Damage (Shāng hán lùn)* and *Essentials from the Golden Cabinet (Jīn guì yào lüè)*, but also the extremely difficult-to-memorize *Divine Husbandman's Classic of the Materia Medica (Shén Nóng běn cǎo jīng)*. Dr. Chen's scholarship and clinical experience was vast. He excelled at treating mishandled cases of cold damage, as well as any other cases that had gone badly. Because he spent a great deal of time making house calls and treating emergency situations, he had little time for writing. He only produced one book, entitled *Thorough Investigations into Medicine (Yī xué tàn yuán)*. Dr. Jiang not only learned the experience of Dr. Chen completely and accurately, he also developed it further.

In those years, Dr. Jiang's students were abundant in the Leshan area, and they followed him in their medical studies, group after group. Everyone was united in their praise for Dr. Jiang. They all spoke of the outstanding training, his high moral virtues, and his vast clinical experience. And yet, nobody stepped forward to do the work of collating and organizing all his experience. At that time, I was still working in a rural hospital in the countryside. One time, while on vacation in Leshan, I learned that Dr. Jiang wanted to write a paper for presentation at a conference on Chinese medicine in Chengdu. However, because of how busy he was in clinic, he had no time to write. This situation aroused my own desire to write.

Dr. Jiang's topic was "The relationship between *Discussion of Cold Damage (Shāng hán lùn)* and warm disease theory." His main intention was to argue for a unification of these two approaches. Ironically, I was firmly opposed to this idea. Nonetheless, I forced myself to strictly follow Dr. Jiang's line of reasoning and write down his thoughts, without interjecting any of my own ideas. Ultimately, this paper led to a contentious debate among the participants at the conference. Dr. Jiang truly appreciated my efforts on his behalf. Not only had I respected him enough to convey his ideas faithfully, but I had also stoutly and generously defended his ideas, even though they ran counter to my own. From this time on, I contentedly became Dr. Jiang's assistant, diligently carrying on his work and organizing the records of his clinical experience. As I gathered testimonials and evidence of his clinical expertise, we published dozens of articles on Chinese medicine.

In fact, I felt very happy and relaxed doing this work for Dr. Jiang. Why? Dr. Jiang was carrying on the work of Dr. Chen. Each time he cured a patient, there was a clearly observable and systematic relationship between "treatment principle, treatment method, formula, and herbs." This relationship particularly highlighted that the selected formula was derived from the method, and that as the correct method emerged, the formula naturally followed. Each time a formula was chosen, not only did it naturally emerge from the treatment principle and method, but there was also a unity between the formula and the herbs. The herbs within the formula never strayed. In other words, if any herbs were added or removed from the formula, there had to be a rationale that could be found in the method and principle.

In looking over the large volume of Dr. Jiang's clinical records, it is clear that he was able to avoid two common mistakes. When using the approach of matching a formula to a pattern, he did not do this mechanically and so avoided the error of "having a formula without [paying attention to the] herbs." When utilizing the approach of differentiating patterns to determine treatment, he was not flippant about his choices and so avoided the error of "having herbs without [a coherent] formula." Because of how conscientious Dr. Jiang was in his work, collating and organizing this type of systematic knowledge did not require much effort on my part.

Furthermore, setting down these theoretical discussions into articles was not difficult, as Dr. Jiang was very eloquent. As soon as we began to discuss questions relating to Chinese medicine, a torrent of words would come out that would unlock profound mysteries through references to the classic texts. He would connect these to modern problems in a way that revealed new ideas. The most difficult part for me was writing quickly enough to keep up with Dr. Jiang's stream of ideas!

ASSISTING IN THE CREATION OF THE "ADVANCED CLASS BY JIANG ER-XUN"

In January 1985, as I arrived at the Leshan City People's Hospital, I was filled with a new sense of purpose. This was the place in which I was helping to establish the class for advanced level students of Jiang Er-Xun, all of whom would be practicing physicians. In my role within the class I had a special status, because not only was I attending, I was also overseeing the administration of the class and participating in the teaching.

Drafting an educational plan

After careful consideration and much thought, I drafted an educational plan for the advanced class in accordance with Dr. Jiang's wishes. The content of these classes would have a primary focus on the work of Zhang Zhong-Jing with background materials from the *Inner Classic (Nèi jīng)*, *Classic of Difficulties (Nàn jīng)*, and *Divine Husbandsman's Classic of the Materia Medica (Shén Nóng běn cǎo jīng)*. These foundational texts were supplemented with famous representative texts from later periods that reflected the strengths of both cold damage theory and warm disease theory. Our goal was to master these texts through comprehensive study in order to make effective use of them in the clinic. The physician-students were asked to follow Dr. Jiang in the clinic, taking notes and gradually accumulating experience. This experience was then tested by them in their own clinics, so that they could learn what was truly valuable. This experience was also used to assess the value of the texts that they were reading, and ultimately they were asked to summarize their own experiences in a systematic fashion.

Students were expected to study theory mainly on their own and then discuss it among themselves. Only after this process could significant or difficult problems be brought to a teacher. When students came up against a difficult problem that exposed a weakness in their prior medical training, extra classes and tutoring were provided.

Students were expected to combine study with clinical practice and they could neglect neither analysis nor memorization. They were asked to take initiative in their studies and to be enthusiastic and creative in their approach to study and reflection. Furthermore, we asked them to be bold in setting forth, analyzing, and answering questions. We insisted on the principles of learning through teaching and of learning through discussion of contentious ideas. We developed a vigorous democracy of learning in which there was a robust and dynamic learning atmosphere that encouraged the development of new ideas.

In the *Posthumous Papers of Master Chu (Chǔ shì yí shū)*, the sixth-century doctor Chu Cheng writes that those who study medicine should "have abundant knowledge of disease," "knowledge of the pulse through many examinations," and "repeatedly use herbs." The Qing-dynasty physician Wang Meng-Ying cautioned students of medicine "not to become a two-legged bookcase." Thus, the educational plan for these classes was "to stand on the shoulders" of those who had come before.

The idea that physicians should "take initiative in their studies and be enthusiastic and creative in their approach to study and reflection" and "be bold in setting forth, analyzing, and answering questions" came from a set of college educational reforms set out by Mao Ze-Dong in 1964. I heard the ideas in his "Remarks at the Spring Festival" *(Chūn jié zhǐ shì)* and from then on, they had remained embedded in my brain.

Taking Charge of Writing Educational Materials

I personally attended to the writing of the educational materials. I always took this job very seriously and I never attempted to fudge things or have others do my work. The collation and organization of these materials continued carefully through many edits, with all of us working hand in hand, until there was nothing left to be corrected. Only then were they submitted for publication.

Hard work does not deter one with a set goal and all these pieces were successful. During a three-year period, four of us worked together to publish more than 50 articles derived from our work collating, organizing, and passing down information from Dr. Jiang. It is worth noting that prior to the establishment of the class of advanced students, none of these physicians had published even a single article. However, because of this experience, some of the outstanding students from that group went on to become highly proficient at writing and publishing articles on Chinese medicine.

I also held an examination of sorts for students who were working on their writing skills. Many of these students had an inferiority complex about their work, because they feared that the quality was poor and that their writings would be ridiculed. In order to overcome these fears, I selected an editorial from a very famous journal of Chinese medicine for their "exam." I told them that although this editorial did not even contain one-thousand characters, it had more than 20 clearly identifiable errors in grammar and punctuation. Their exam was to go through and correct all these errors. Doing this work opened their eyes and relieved them of their sense of inferiority.

Conclusion

The great Tang-dynasty poet Lu You remarked that "if you wish to learn poetry, place your efforts outside of poetry." I don't see how this is any different for those studying medicine. I failed to succeed at my original university specialty of political economics and yet the core curriculum of that study, especially *Das Kapital* by Karl Marx, provided me with a foundation in the humanities, philosophy, and science. My efforts and studies in those domains provided me with a key to unlock the treasure trove of knowledge within the field of Chinese medicine.

During the time when I was reaching a higher level in my work, the structure of my intellectual knowledge and my mode of thinking provided me, consciously or unconsciously, with a truly unique vantage point. I was able to view the study of Chinese medicine through multiple lenses and appreciate the beauty within. Not only was I relatively objective and clear-eyed in my views, but I had a real appreciation for my studies, even to the point of sometimes feeling intoxicated.

The Ming-dynasty philosopher Hong Ying-Ming said, "Mountain scenery viewed through the rain has a fresh beauty; listening quietly to the tolling of bells at night, the sound is especially clear and seems to travel especially far." As I have traversed the rugged path of my career in Chinese medicine, I have worked tirelessly, without any feelings of fatigue or occupational burnout, because the long journey has had "a fresh beauty" and "the sound is especially clear and seems to travel especially far." In other words, like Su Dong-Po (whose hometown of Meishan I passed going to Chengdu), while I can "look back at the desolate places [challenges and hardships] that I have passed through," I do not feel any resentment or regret, but only an ever-increasing sense of my own good fortune.

CHAPTER 1

Disorders of the Qi, Blood, and Body Fluids

1.1.1 **Blood patterns**

A three-year case of recurrent hemoptysis that has worsened in the last month

A formula that has been pounded and tempered myriad times

經過千錘百鍊的方劑

■ CASE HISTORY

Patient: *39-year-old male*

The patient suffered from pulmonary tuberculosis ten years prior to our intake and had been treated successfully with an anti-consumption regimen. Over the last three years he expectorated a small amount of fresh blood or sputum streaked with blood whenever he overworked or had a cold. Multiple examinations have ruled out a recurrence of pulmonary tuberculosis and is it suspected that he has bronchiectasis.

Twenty-eight days ago, after a domestic dispute, the patient became furious, drank several glasses of liquor and then fell into a deep sleep. In the middle of the night he woke up, had an attack of coughing, and suddenly noticed the taste of blood in his throat. Soon afterwards he expectorated a mouthful of blood and by daybreak had expectorated blood three times for a total of about 400ml (about 1.3 cups). He was promptly taken to the hospital.

The patient underwent examination and testing at the hospital at which time bronchiectasis was considered the most likely diagnosis. He was given hemostatic, anti-inflammatory, and antibiotic drugs by the Western medical doctors along with intravenous fluids and a blood transfusion. He was in intensive care for seven days during which time he continued to frequently expectorate small amounts of fresh blood.

He was then treated by traditional Chinese medical doctors with more than ten packets of Gentian Decoction to Drain the Liver *(lóng dǎn xiè gān tāng)*, Rhinoceros Horn and Rehmannia Decoction *(xī jiǎo dì huáng tāng)*—substituting Bubali Cornu *(shuǐ niú jiǎo)* for the *xī jiǎo* normally used in the formula—combined with Lily Bulb Decoction to Preserve the Metal *(bǎi hé gù jīn tāng)*. While this treatment reduced the frequency of expectoration, still every two or three days the patient would expectorate about 100ml of blood once or twice.

INTAKE EXAMINATION
DATE: July 21, 1984

Before each attack of hemoptysis, the patient reported feeling a rush of hot qi flushing up into his chest and throat. This was accompanied by expectoration of fresh-red blood, a slight cough and occasional expectoration of blood-streaked sputum. His mouth was dry and he preferred cold drinks, his breath had a dirty smell, and he had constipation. We observed a thin, red tongue that lacked moisture and had a thin, yellow coating with scant fluids, and a wiry, long, and slightly rapid pulse.

DIFFERENTIATION OF PATTERNS AND DISCUSSION OF TREATMENT

PHYSICIAN A   Hemoptysis is called coughing up of blood in Chinese medicine and refers to the coughing up of either blood-streaked sputum or fresh-red blood. Since the blood emanates from the lungs, the disorder is thought to stem from injury to the collaterals of the Lung.

Contemporary Chinese medical textbooks generally attribute this disorder to one of three pattern types and direct treatment accordingly:

- Dryness and heat damaging the Lung: a modified version of Mulberry Leaf and Apricot Kernel Decoction *(sāng xìng tāng)* is used to calm the collaterals and arrest bleeding.

- Liver fire accosting the Lung: Drain the White Powder *(xiè bái sǎn)* and Indigo and Clamshell Powder *(dài gé sǎn)*[1] are used to clear the Liver, drain the Lung, cool the blood, and stop bleeding.

- Lung heat from yin deficiency: Lily Bulb Decoction to Preserve the Metal *(bǎi hé gù jīn tāng)* is used to enrich the yin, moisten the Lung, calm the collaterals, and stop bleeding.

So, does this case fit into one of the above patterns?

....

1. This formula is made up simply of the substances Indigo naturalis *(qīng dài)* and Meretricis/Cyclinae Concha *(gé qiào)* at a 1:10 ratio.

DR. YU   This patient certainly displays many manifestations of excess heat. However, given that he has had recurrent hemoptysis for three years that has worsened in the last month, and that this has continued despite repeated usage of Chinese and Western medicine, one must consider that a root deficiency underlies the etiology.

Let us carefully examine his symptoms. He states that before attacks of hemoptysis he feels a rush of hot qi flushing up into his chest and throat from the lower abdomen. This obviously is counterflow ascent of Penetrating vessel qi. Chapter 60 of the *Basic Questions (Sū wèn)* states, "When the Penetrating vessel suffers illness it gives rise to counterflow qi and internal cramping." The Penetrating vessel connects down to the *shào yīn* and reaches up to the *yáng míng*. When the yin and essence of *shào yīn* are exhausted and deficient, fluids wither and lose containment. It is difficult for the Penetrating vessel qi to calmly stay in its chamber and it shifts and rises in counterflow, carrying Stomach qi with it, and it also rises in counterflow and collides with the Lung qi.

Therefore, because the Penetrating vessel qi is unsteady and rises in counterflow, we can infer that the *shào yīn* is exhausted and deficient.

Furthermore, the patient's tongue was red, thin, and lacking in moisture. This is also a sign of exhaustion of the yin and thin fluids.

One way of looking at the wiry, long pulse is based on the work of the Ming-dynasty author Li Shi-Cai (also known as Li Zhong-Zi) who said, "Straight up and straight down is a Penetratiing [vessel] pulse; its travels straight up and straight down again and again until it [stretches out and] becomes long." From this we can see that wiry and long describes a pulse that is reflecting pathology of the Penetrating vessel.

In sum, we can surmise that the primary pathodynamic in this case of hemoptysis is exhaustion and deficiency of the *sháo yīn* yin essence, surplus *yáng míng* qi and fire, and upward counterflow of Penetrating vessel qi. This is a complex presentation with a deficient root and an excess branch.

Treatment and Outcome

Having determined that this disorder is due to deficiency of the yin essence of *sháo yīn*, surplus *yáng míng* qi and fire, and counterflow ascent of Penetrating (vessel) qi, the treatment principle should be to enrich and nourish the *shào yīn*, clear and drain the *yáng míng*, calm the Penetrating vessel and direct counterflow ascent downwards.

Rehmanniae Radix praeparata *(shú dì huáng)*	30g
Untreated Gypsum fibrosum *(shēng shí gāo)*	30g
Achyranthis bidentatae Radix *(niú xī)*	15g
Ophiopogonis Radix *(mài mén dōng)*	15g
Anemarrhenae Rhizoma *(zhī mǔ)*	6g
Scutellariae Radix *(huáng qín)*	10g
Polygoni cuspidati Rhizoma *(hǔ zhàng)*	30g
Untreated Haematitum *(shēng dài zhě shí)*	4.5g
Untreated Euryales Semen *(shēng qiàn shí)*	12g

Instructions: three packets

SECOND VISIT: For five days after the last visit the patient did not experience any upward flushing of hot qi and had no episodes of hemoptysis. His bowel movements became smooth and his experience of dry mouth and bad breath declined. He still had a slight cough and his sputum was occasionally blood-streaked.

We modified the above formula by removing Untreated Haematitum *(shēng dài zhě shí)*, Untreated Euryales Semen *(shēng qiàn shí)*, and Polygoni cuspidati Rhizoma *(hǔ zhàng)* and adding Agrimoniae Herba *(xiān hè cǎo)* 30g, Imperatae Rhizoma *(bái máo gēn)* 30g, and Nelumbinis Nodus rhizomatis *(ǒu jié)* 15g. We prescribed six packets.

THIRD VISIT: During the two weeks since his first visit the patient had no hemoptysis. The slight cough with blood-streaked sputum was also absent. His tongue and pulse were, at this time, unremarkable.

The prescription was changed to an unmodified Decoction to Patch the Collaterals and Vessels (絡補管湯 *bǔ luò bu guǎn tāng*), a formula designed by the well-known early 20th-century physician, Zhang Xi-Chun:

untreated Fossilia Ossis Mastodi *(shēng lóng gǔ)* 30g

untreated Ostreae Concha *(shēng mǔ lì)* 30g

Corni Fructus *(shān zhū yú)*... 30g

Notoginseng Radix *(sān qī)*... 6g

Instructions: powdered and taken 3g twice a day chased with the strained decoction.
15 packets prescribed

The patient had a follow-up visit two years later and stated that he had experienced no recurrence of hemoptysis.

Disease	Primary symptoms	Differential diagnosis	Treatment method	Formula
Hemoptysis	Recurrent expectoration of blood	Exhausted and deficient *shào yīn* yin essence, surplus *yáng míng* qi and fire, upward counterflow of Penetrating vessel qi. The root is deficiency and the branch is excess.	Enrich the *shào yīn*, clear and drain the *yáng míng*, calm flushing and direct counterflow downward	Augmented Jade Woman Decoction *(yù nǚ jiān)*

REFLECTIONS AND CLARIFICATIONS

PHYSICIAN B   Contemporary textbooks divide hemoptysis into three types, as noted above, and do not include anything like the deficiency and excess complex described in this case of hemoptysis treated with an augmented form of Jade Woman Decoction *(yù nǚ jiān)*. In the textbooks, this formula is used for epistaxis that pertains to intensely blazing Stomach heat. However, since this condition pertains to excess heat, to match the condition correctly, the Rehmanniae Radix praeparata *(shú dì huáng)* in the formula should be replaced with Rehmanniae Radix *(shēng dì huáng)*.

In this case you are using an augmented Jade Woman Decoction *(yù nǚ jiān)* to treat hemoptysis where the patient coughs up bright-red blood and has a set of excess heat signs such as a dry mouth, bad breath, and constipation. You not only don't change Rehmanniae Radix praeparata *(shú dì huáng)* to its untreated form, but raise its dosage to 30g and add Euryales Semen *(qiàn shí)* to benefit the Kidneys and secure the essence. What are the reasons for this?

DR. YU   I selected augmented Jade Woman Decoction *(yù nǚ jiān)* to use the original formula's Untreated Gypsum fibrosum *(shēng shí gāo)* and Anemarrhenae Rhizoma *(zhī mǔ)* to clear and drain *yáng míng* fire; Rehmanniae Radix praeparata *(shú dì huáng)* to enrich and replenish insufficient *shào yīn* essence; with Ophiopogonis Radix *(mài mén dōng)* to nourish the yin and clear the Lung; and in order to enable the mutual generation of metal and water and insure that the source springs of essence are not exhausted. Achyranthis bidentatae Radix *(niú xī)* guides the heat downward and out of the body.

Untreated Euryales Semen *(shēng qiàn shí)* is included to restrain the flushing of qi, along with untreated Haematitum *(shēng dài zhě shí)* to direct Stomach qi downward and subdue flushing, Scutellariae Radix *(huáng qín)* to drain fire and stop bleeding, and Polygoni cuspidati Rhizoma *(hǔ zhàng)* to drain heat and unblock the bowels. These modifications extend the reach of the original formula.

PHYSICIAN B   Do you apply Jade Woman Decoction *(yù nǚ jiān)* to the treatment of many disease patterns that give rise to ascendant flooding of blood?

DR. YU   Speaking frankly, clinically I am not fond of Zhang Jing-Yue's formulas, but there is a special place in my heart for Jade Woman Decoction *(yù nǚ jiān)*, and I often employ it. The credit for this goes to my teacher, Jiang Er-Xun.

All of you know that while Dr. Jiang liked to use classic formulas, he was not at all dismissive of formulas from later periods. Through extensive use of these formulas he discovered that they could be quite effective and on a level with the formulas of Zhang Zhong-Jing. Jade Woman Decoction *(yù nǚ jiān)* is one of the post-classic formulas that he appreciated.

He liked to modify this formula, using it to treat a variety of patterns including *shào yīn* insufficiency with *yáng míng* surplus that results in headaches, eye pain, tooth pain, sore throat, and even vomiting of blood or nosebleeds. He frequently obtained excellent results.

Regarding this formula, Zhang Jing-Yue said:

> It treats exhausted water with overabundant fire with all six pulses being floating, overflowing, slippery, and large. The *shào yīn* is insufficient and the *yáng míng* has surplus [this manifests as] irritability-heat with dryness and thirst, headache, toothache, and blood loss, all of which the formula treats with miraculous effect.

Of course, we should take the "miraculous effect" statement with a grain of salt and rely on clinical experience to guide us.

PHYSICIAN B   If understood like this, then the pointed criticisms of Jade Woman Decoction *(yù nǚ jiān)* by Chen Xiu-Yuan should not be taken as gospel.

DR. YU   They are definitely not to be taken as gospel. In Chen Xiu-Yuan's *A Critique of [Zhang] Jing-Yue's New Formulas (Jǐng-Yuè xīn fāng biān)*, he makes this pointed criticism of Jade Woman Decoction *(yù nǚ jiān)*:

> [Zhang] Zhong-Jing used Gypsum fibrosum *(shí gāo)* to clear the middle as in the two decoctions White Tiger Decoction *(bái hǔ tāng)* and Lophatherum and Gypsum Decoction *(zhú yè shí gāo tāng)*; he used Gypsum fibrosum *(shí gāo)* to dispel pathogens as in the two decoctions Major Bluegreen Dragon Decoction

(dà qīng lóng tāng) and Maidservant from Yue's Decoction *(Yuè bì tāng)*; and he used Gypsum fibrosum *(shí gāo)* as something that could be added or subtracted in the two decoctions Minor Bluegreen Dragon Decoction *(xiǎo qīng lóng tāng)* and Cocculus Decoction *(mù fáng jǐ tāng)*. All these usages are ingenious. When [Zhang] Jing-Yue uses [Gypsum fibrosum *(shí gāo)*] with Rehmanniae Radix praeparata *(shú dì huáng)* and Achyranthis bidentatae Radix *(niú xī)*, he is totally discarding the classic methods.

This implies that because [Zhang] Zhong-Jing never used Gypsum fibrosum *(shí gāo)* together with Rehmanniae Radix praeparata *(shú dì huáng)* and Achyranthis bidentatae Radix *(niú xī)*, people later should never ever do so. And if one ever did use them together, this would be disrespectful to [Zhang] Zhong-Jing and tantamount to completely discarding classic methods. This obviously goes too far in adoration of the classics and adulation of the ancients.

Chen Xiu-Yuan also mysteriously said:

> The formula is named Jade Woman Decoction, which displays both self-aggrandizement and a portent of ill fortune. In the south of Fujian there is a custom that friends and relatives burn votive candles to the dead and always write on the candles, "The Golden Boy (金童 *jīn tóng*) goes and guides [the soul] while the Jade Girl (玉女 *yù nǚ*) comes and receives [the soul]." [2] This comment reveals Chen Xiu-Yuan's belief in superstition!

Even further from the norm is his sharing of his personal experience to warn the people of the world, "With my own eyes I've seen that when I've given this decoction not a one has not matched this portent. Beware of it, beware!" He is implying that taking Jade Woman Decoction *(yù nǚ jiān)* would lead to having the Golden Boy and Jade Girl taking you to the netherworld.

This is certainly not correct, but we should consider when we talk about this issue that in the days when Chen Xiu-Yuan was writing *A Critique of [Zhang] Jing-Yue's New Formulas (Jǐng-Yuè xīn fāng biān)*, aside from his adoration of the classics and adulation of the ancients, there was another important reason he wrote in this manner. He felt that the formulas constructed by the esteemed ancients should usually not be changed, as every such constructed formula (especially the classic formulas of Zhang Zhong-Jing) had been pounded and tempered myriad times and had only taken their final form after having been proved to be highly effective. Contrarily, Zhang Jing-Yue seemingly constructed formulas with ease, and in a very short time had created so many formulas that he could categorize them as "The Eight Tactical Arrays of New Formulas." Of these, how many had really been pounded and tempered myriad times?

We can see the truth of this point in a modern context as new formulas and 'secret' formulas spring up like mushrooms after a rain shower, one after another. Some appear in the news media with great fanfare and provide truly wondrous descriptions. Yet of all these formulas, how many really have any evidence of being clinically effective? Therefore, if we employ this perspective, Chen Xiu-Yuan's *A Critique of [Zhang] Jing-Yue's New Formulas (Jǐng-Yuè xīn fāng biān)* has still not lost its practical import.

....

2. The Golden Boy and Jade Girl are the assistants to advanced Daoist sages and are often pictured standing next to Guan Yin.

PHYSICIAN A   By the third visit the patient had not expectorated blood for half of a month. According to the conventions set down by the early modern physician Tang Zong-Hai, once any bleeding has stopped, the next steps should be to reduce stasis, calm the blood, and tonify the blood. You only use Decoction to Patch the Collaterals and Vessels *(bǔ luò bu guǎn tāng)* as a treatment at this stage and yet there were no relapses for at least two years after taking it. What is the reasoning behind this?

DR. YU   Zhang Xi-Chun designed Decoction to Patch the Collaterals and Vessels *(bǔ luò bu guǎn tāng)* to treat "coughing or spitting up of blood that has persisted for a long time without getting better." His use of herbs has its singular aspects. He stated:

> Fossilia Ossis Mastodi *(lóng gǔ)*, Ostreae Concha *(mǔ lì)*, and Corni Fructus *(shān zhū yú)* restrain and bind while also having the power to open up and connect. Therefore, they can tonify the Lung collaterals and the gastric blood vessels to utilize their ability to stop bleeding while not making the mistake of stopping it too precipitously, which can lead to the problem of residual stasis. Furthermore, the ability of the assistant Notoginseng Radix *(sān qī)* to transform putrefaction and generate new flesh leads to a smooth recovery of the injured areas. As its nature is to excel at regulating the blood, it is a wonderful product for treatment of spitting up or vomiting of blood.

According to Zhang's explanation, this formula is not only useful for stopping bleeding, but also has the functions of reducing stasis and calming and tonifying the blood. I like to use this formula when treating disorders involving chronic bleeding. It also treats acute bleeding disorders and is therefore ideal for treating bleeding from accidental injuries and trauma. I have used it successfully in treating several acute situations of this type.

PHYSICIAN A   I have a supplementary question. 'Hemoptysis' is a Western medical term; in Chinese medicine this is usually called 'coughing blood' instead of 'hemoptysis.' Is there really any difference between these two terms?

DR. YU   There is a difference, although many doctors confuse the two terms. Even the famous late nineteenth-century doctor Tang Zong-Hai stated that "'Hemoptysis' is streaks of blood in sputum."

According to the *Sea of Words (Cí hǎi)*, a well-respected encyclopedic dictionary, the character 咯 [pronounced *luò* in this case], which is nowadays translated as hemoptysis, when used as a verb means to retch or vomit. It does not carry the meaning "to cough." The *Concise Dictionary of Chinese Medicine (Jiǎn míng zhōng yī cí diǎn)* explains the term 咯血 *(luò xuè)* [translated here as hemoptysis] as "indicating that there is a bloody taste in the throat and expectoration produces blood or freshly clotted blood … mostly due to yin deficiency with exuberant fire or dry heat in the Lung." Its explanation of coughing of blood (咳血 *ké xuè*) is "production of blood during coughing. There may be blood-streaked sputum or pure blood. … It is mostly due to an externally-contracted wind pathogen not being released or transforming into heat or dryness and injuring the collaterals of the Lung, or from Liver fire accosting the Lung."

From a clinical perspective, the differentiation of the etiology and pathodynamic of hemoptysis and coughing of blood may seem forced, yet there is a difference in their presentations. There may not be a clear coughing activity in hemoptysis, while in coughing of blood, the blood must appear because of the coughing.

An ancient physician who explained this difference very clearly was Zhang Jing-Yue, who said, "In hemoptysis [blood] will come out with slight expectoration from the throat. This is not like the intense use of energy seen with coughing of blood." This description is correct. We need to pay attention to this difference when recording cases.

1.1.2 Bleeding

Three years of recurrent urethral bleeding that has worsened in the last two months

Local and systemic pathodynamics

局部病機與整體病機

■ CASE HISTORY

Patient: *35-year-old male*

Thirteen years ago the patient bruised his genitals, which led to severe urethral bleeding that ceased after emergency treatment. This condition recurred one time five years ago, but recurrences have become more frequent over the last three years. Bleeding occurs every time the patient gets chilled, becomes overtired, or has intercourse. Fortunately, the combined use of Chinese and Western drugs leads to a gradual cessation of the bleeding.

Two months ago, after a succession of late nights, the patient suffered copious urethral bleeding with continual dripping throughout the night. Out-patient treatment was unsuccessful, and he was admitted to the surgical ward. He was treated with intravenous fluids, blood transfusions, and anti-infectious and symptom-based treatments, which reduced the amount of bleeding. He concurrently took more than 40 packets of Chinese herbs but the bleeding still did not cease.

Examination of the patient's chart revealed that most of the tailored herb formulas he had been given aimed at clearing heat, cooling the blood, transforming stasis and stopping bleeding. They were based on such formulas as Small Thistle Drink *(xiǎo jì yǐn zi)*, Powder for Five Types of Painful Urinary Dribbling *(wǔ lín sǎn)*, and Rhinoceros Horn and Rehmannia Decoction *(xī jiǎo dì huáng tāng)*. However, the most recent formula was a decoction version of Kidney Qi Pill from the *Golden Cabinet (jīn guì shèn qì wán)* with the addition of Achyranthis bidentatae Radix *(niú xī)* to guide fire to return to its source.

INTAKE EXAMINATION
DATE: December 6, 1985

Fresh blood was slowly oozing from the patient's urethra (unrelated to the passage of urine), or dripping out, or exuding in string-like globules. The patient experiences 4-6 episodes of painless bleeding per 24 hours, each time discharging 2-5ml of blood.

During his time in the hospital, the patient underwent numerous examinations, including ultrasound, cystoscopy, and x-rays, and had several tests of his entire urogenital system. No lesion of any kind was found. There was no way to make a definitive biomedical diagnosis.

The patient's complexion lacked luster, he appeared fatigued, was short of breath, had adequate food intake, slightly loose stools, a pale, purplish tongue with a thin, white coating, and a wiry, moderate pulse that lacked strength when pressure was applied.

DIFFERENTIATION OF PATTERN AND DISCUSSION OF TREATMENT

PHYSICIAN A   In the final analysis what disease has caused this case of urethral bleeding? Specifically, how can one firmly establish a diagnosis in this case?

DR. YU   It seems as if no disease like this can be found in Chinese medicine texts. While, when the patient urinates, naturally there is blood mixed in with his urine, blood also seeps from his urethral opening when he is not urinating, so this problem cannot be considered in the category of blood in the urine (尿血 *niào xuè*). If it cannot be considered a form of blood in the urine, it therefore cannot be considered a type of painful urinary dribbling with bleeding (血淋 *xuè lín*); this thought is reinforced by the fact that there is not a hint of pain in this patient's presentation.

Western medicine also cannot make a diagnosis here, despite having performed numerous examinations and tests using modern equipment, none of which found any lesions.

If we must choose a disease name for diagnostic purposes, for the time being we can use recurrent urethral bleeding.

PHYSICIAN A   This is a case of recurrent urethral bleeding for three years that has worsened over the last two months. Both Chinese and Western medicines have been used repeatedly, yet the bleeding has not stopped. Analysis based on the patient's complexion, which lacks luster, and his fatigued appearance, shortness of breath, loose stools, pale, purplish tongue with a thin, white coating, and a pulse that is wiry and moderate but disappears on pressure leads to the conclusion that the pathodynamic is deficient qi failing to contain blood.

What is difficult for me to understand is why, given this clear pattern of symptoms, the previous doctors didn't put two and two together, but continued to use heat-clearing, yin-enriching, and blood-cooling herbs and formulas for such a long time.

DR. YU   Although the patient had the complete set of signs and symptoms indicative of deficient qi failing to contain the blood when he came to see me, we do not know if this was the case when his problems began. What is considered a pattern in Chinese medicine is the singular essence of a particular contradiction that occurs at a given stage in the development of disease.[3] Therefore the word *stage* must be considered. To me:

....

3. *Translators' note:* This language comes from Mao's essay, "On Contradiction" (矛盾論 *Máo dùn lùn*).

1. Perhaps the beginning stage of this patient's increased severity of urethral bleeding did pertain to chaotic movement of hot blood, so the previous physicians appropriately used formulas and herbs that cleared heat, cooled the blood, and stanched bleeding.

2. A problem developed after herbs to clear heat, cool blood and stanch bleeding were employed in too large a dosage and for too long a time. This injured the qi, damaged the blood and cooled the collaterals giving rise to congealing and stasis. The pattern then gradually changed and became one of deficient qi failing to contain blood.

3. The previous physicians had already acknowledged their mistake and that is why the last formula prescribed was Kidney Qi Pill *(shèn qì wán)* plus Achyranthis bidentatae Radix *(niú xī)* to lead the fire back to its source. This change clearly indicates their recognition of the issue.

Isn't this a more objective way of evaluating the merits and faults of the previous physicians' approach?

PHYSICIAN A   If the doctors had obstinately continued to wrongly use herbs and formulas that cleared heat, cooled the blood, and stopped bleeding, what do you think would have happened?

DR. YU   The body's qi would have followed the blood and flowed from the body; this would have resulted in a state of abandonment!

The preliminary understanding, based on a synthetic analysis of the history, course of treatment, and presenting symptoms, is that of injury to the collaterals and vessels of the genitals leading to qi failing to contain blood. We tested this with a combination of Decoction to Tonify the Collaterals and Repair the [Blood] Vessels *(bǔ luò bǔ guǎntāng)* and Tonify the Middle to Augment the Qi Decoction *(bǔ zhōng yì qì tāng)*:

untreated Fossilia Ossis Mastodi *(lóng gǔ)*	30g
untreated Ostreae Concha *(mǔ lì)*	30g
Corni Fructus *(shān zhū yú)*	30g
Notoginseng Radix *(sān qī)*	[3g per dose] 6g
[ground and chased with strained decoction]	
Astragali Radix *(huáng qí)*	30g
Codonopsis Radix *(dǎng shēn)*	15g
Atractylodis macrocephalae Rhizoma *(bái zhú)*	15g
Glycyrrhizae Radix praeparata *(zhì gān cǎo)*	6g
Cimicifugae Rhizoma *(shēng má)*	6g
Bupleuri Radix *(chái hú)*	6g
Angelicae sinensis Radix *(dāng guī)*	10g
Citri reticulatae Pericarpium *(chén pí)*	10g

After taking two packets the patient reported no seepage of blood during the day and only twice at night, with a marked reduction in the volume of seepage.

I needed to travel out of town, so the patient was seen by an old Chinese doctor to whom he showed the above prescription. His line of thinking about the case was in accord with ours and so he continued along the same lines, but made some modifications to the ingredients:

Cirsii Herba *(xiǎo jì)* 30g
Nelumbinis Nodus rhizomatis *(ǒu jié)* 15g
Rubiae Radix *(qiàn cǎo gēn)* 15g
Rehmanniae Radix *(shēng dì huáng)* 30g
Notoginseng Radix *(sān qī)* .... [3g per dose] 6g
    [ground and chased with strained decoction]
Astragali Radix *(huáng qí)* 30g
Codonopsis Radix *(dǎng shēn)* 15g
Atractylodis macrocephalae Rhizoma *(bái zhú)* 15g
Glycyrrhizae Radix praeparata *(zhì gān cǎo)* 6g
Cimicifugae Rhizoma *(shēng má)* 6g
Bupleuri Radix *(chái hú)* 6g
Angelicae sinensis Radix *(dāng guī)* 10g
Citri reticulatae Pericarpium *(chén pí)* 10g

Five packets were prescribed, but after taking three packets the bleeding increased, so he stopped taking this prescription and went to see a doctor who combined Chinese and Western medicines. This doctor thought the problem was that the long-term urethral bleeding had damaged the capillaries in the corpus spongiosum of the penis and therefore prescribed Three-Seed Decoction *(sān rén tāng)* along with a large dosage of Phellodendri Cortex *(huáng bǎi)*, Plantaginis Herba *(chē qián cǎo)*, and Imperatae Rhizoma *(bái máo gēn)*. Five packets were prescribed.

After taking just two packets, the patient began bleeding both day and night, with the nighttime bleeding being especially profuse. He understandably didn't dare continue with these herbs. He was so desperate that he almost panicked. When he heard that I had returned to town, he rushed over to see me and explained all the setbacks that had occurred.

After observing the patient's pulse and the rest of his presentation, it was clear to me that the first formula I had used should be employed again, with the addition of Special Pill to Transform Blood *(huà xuè dān)*, a formula developed by the early 20th-century physician, Zhang Xi-Chun.

calcined Ophicalcitum *(duàn huā ruì shí)* 10g
Notoginseng Radix *(sān qī)* 6g
Crinis carbonisatus *(xuè yú tàn)* 3g

These three substances were to be ground into a fine powder and taken in two doses with warm water twice a day, morning and evening.

After taking five packets of both formulas, the patient's urethral bleeding had stopped completely. He was then urged to take ten more packets of the original formula to secure the effects. On follow-up a year later, there had been no recurrence of urethral bleeding.

REFLECTIONS AND CLARIFICATIONS

PHYSICIAN B   In the beginning your use of Tonify the Middle to Augment the Qi Decoction *(bǔ zhōng yì qì tāng)* matched the presentation. Why did you additionally use

Disease	Primary symptoms	Differential diagnosis	Treatment method	Formula
Urethral bleeding	Recurrent seepage of blood from the urethra along with lusterless complexion, fatigue, and shortness of breath	Injury and damage to the collaterals and vessels of the genitals; qi not containing blood	Tonify qi and contain blood; tonify the collaterals and repair the blood vessels	Decoction to Tonify the Collaterals and Repair the [Blood] Vessels (bǔ luò bǔ guǎn tāng) with Tonify the Middle to Augment the Qi Decoction (bǔ zhōng yì qì tāng)

Fossilia Ossis Mastodi *(lóng gǔ)*, Ostreae Concha *(mǔ lì)*, Corni Fructus *(shān zhū yú)*, and Notoginseng Radix *(sān qī)*?

DR. YU   A more accurate description would be "collectively use" as opposed to "additionally use." These four ingredients make up a formula devised by Zhang Xi-Chun called Decoction to Tonify the Collaterals and Repair the [Blood] Vessels *(bǔ luò bǔ guǎn tāng)*. In his *Essays on Medicine Esteeming the Chinese and Respecting the Western (Yī xúe zhōng zhōng cān xī lù)*, Zhang says that this formula was originally intended to "treat long-term coughing or vomiting of blood." He further wrote that:

> Zhang Jing-Yue stated that, "Over time, coughing will break open the collaterals at the opening of the lungs, such that the person will cough up blood." Westerners say that when the blood vessels in the stomach are damaged and ruptured, the person will vomit blood. Fossilia Ossis Mastodi *(lóng gǔ)*, Ostreae Concha *(mǔ lì)*, and Corni Fructus *(shān zhū yú)* all have restraining and binding natures, while at the same time they can open up and remove obstacles. In this way, they are able to tonify the collaterals of the lungs and the blood vessels of the stomach and function to stop bleeding without leading to the dangers inherent in overly abrupt blood stanching, such as the development of stasis. With the help of Notoginseng Radix *(sān qī)*'s ability to transform putrid [flesh] and generate new [flesh], areas that have been injured and damaged can easily heal.

While this case does not involve coughing or vomiting of blood, this passage did serve as an inspiration to me. The patient suffered trauma to his genital area thirteen years ago, leading to serious urethral bleeding. Five years ago, there was another incident, and for the last three years attacks have been rather frequent. This has been going on a long time! The repeated use of Chinese and Western medicines has been unable to entirely stop the bleeding, so perhaps there has been some damage and breakage of the collaterals and vessels of the genitals.

Zhang stated that this formula can mend broken collaterals in the lung and stomach; he didn't say that it could mend broken collaterals and vessels in the genital area. But if you think about it, both conditions are due to broken collaterals, so there is no difference at all in the mechanism. There was no harm in learning from his experience and trying out this approach.

Tonify the Middle to Augment the Qi Decoction *(bǔ zhōng yì qì tāng)* by itself only tonifies the qi and contains blood, it is unable to tonify the collaterals or repair the vessels. Without mending the areas that have been damaged, it is difficult to entirely stop the bleeding.

PHYSICIAN B   In this instance, the pathodynamic has two parts, not just one:

1. collaterals and vessels that are broken

2. qi not containing the blood

DR. YU   Correct! The injured and broken collaterals and vessels are the local pathodynamic while qi not containing the blood is the systemic pathodynamic. Becoming good at putting local and systemic pathodynamics together to form a comprehensive concept is an essential skill for clinicians.

PHYSICIAN B   That is why it isn't at all strange that there was a substantial increase in bleeding when Decoction to Tonify the Collaterals and Repair the [Blood] Vessels *(bǔ luò bǔ guǎn tāng)* was removed from the prescription and a group of substances were added to cool the blood and stop bleeding.

PHYSICIAN C   During the patient's second visit with you, in addition to the decoction, you added the powder Ophicalcitum *(huā ruì shí)*, Notoginseng Radix *(sān qī)*, and Crinis carbonisatus *(xuè yú tàn)*. Weren't you concerned that this could have led to blood stasis?

DR. YU   I was indeed concerned about the danger of blood stasis and that is why I added those three substances, which are together known as Special Pill to Transform Blood *(huà xuè dān)*. Blood stasis develops when there is prolonged damage to collaterals and vessels. Similarly, cooling, when overdone, leads to congealing and binding in the collaterals and vessels, which exacerbates the stasis and causes it to become more deeply rooted.

Therefore, when thinking of which decoction to use during the first visit, I was afraid that the strength of the herbs would be insufficient to fully address the situation. I turned the problem over in my mind and thought of Special Pill to Transform Blood *(huà xuè dān)*. This is a formula developed by Zhang Xi-Chun. He originally described it as a formula that "treats coughing up of blood and also treats vomiting [of blood] and nosebleeds, regulates static blood, and also addresses blood in the urine or stools." Since, in this case, I used the effects of Decoction to Tonify the Collaterals and Repair the [Blood] Vessels *(bǔ luò bǔ guǎn tāng)* to good end, I could also try this formula, hoping that together they would transform the static blood in the collaterals and vessels of the genitals.

As to whether there is a danger of promoting blood stasis with this formula, Zhang Xi-Chun himself discussed this in detail:

> Most doctors regard Notoginseng Radix *(sān qī)* as a strong medicine for alleviating vomiting of blood and nosebleeds and say that it should not be used lightly. This is incorrect. Notoginseng Radix *(sān qī)* and Ophicalcitum *(huā ruì shí)* are both sage-like medicines that stop bleeding as well as sage-like medicines that transform blood [stasis]. They can transform static blood without damaging new blood. When used to treat vomiting of blood and nosebleeds, there are no post-treatment ill effects. I base this on much experience, so I dare to say it with certainty. … Now, regarding Crinis carbonisatus *(xuè yú tàn)*, its ability to transform static blood is less than that of Ophicalcitum *(huā ruì shí)* and Notoginseng

Radix *(sān qī)*, but its power to tonify the blood is greater. Hair is originally produced from the blood of the human body, so it can give back what was transformed. After it has been charred through calcination, it also can stanch bleeding.

PHYSICIAN C   From this case of urethral bleeding I have come to realize that when treating bleeding, one needs to have an open-minded approach to choosing herbs and formulas and be skilled in drawing from the distinctive experiences of famous physicians.

DR. YU   It is important that while scrupulously abiding by the ancient adage to "use herbs like soldiers, do not lightly deploy them," you don't tie yourself up in knots, but rather grasp any opportunity to take advantage of the situations you encounter to see what can be verified in the clinic. In this way we can expand the scope of efficacy of formulas and herbs.

PHYSICIAN D   I have a supplementary question: Can Decoction to Tonify the Collaterals and Repair the [Blood] Vessels *(bǔ luò bǔ guǎn tāng)* truly treat long-term coughing or vomiting of blood?

DR. YU   I have used an augmented combination of Decoction to Tonify the Collaterals and Repair the [Blood] Vessels *(bǔ luò bǔ guǎn tāng)* and Jade Woman Decoction *(yù nǚ jiān)* to treat several cases of hemoptysis from bronchiectasis. It was very effective. I don't know if it is useful for treating vomiting of blood.

1.2 **Phlegm patterns**

Severe phlegm

Like a fish drinking water, one knows if it is cold or warm [4]

如魚飲水，冷緩自知

■ CASE HISTORY

Patient: *51-year-old female*

Seven days after having her gallbladder removed the patient imprudently became chilled and developed a pulmonary infection. She experienced aversion to cold, high fever, cough with tightness upon breathing, and a hacking cough with clogged and congested, turbid sputum.

The allopathic doctors diagnosed her with bronchial pneumonia (we did not receive the imaging and blood reports). The patient received intravenous fluids, antibiotics, and supportive therapies. She was also given three packets of combined Ephedra, Apricot Kernel,

....

4. This saying, which emphasizes the uniqueness and practical utility of one's own experience, comes from *A History of Pillars (Tīng shǐ* 程史*)*, a collection of stories about the Song era written by Yue Ke 岳珂 in the 13th century.

Gypsum, and Licorice Decoction *(má xìng shí gān tāng)* and Honeysuckle and Forsythia Powder *(yín qiáo sǎn)*. The patient's chills and fever declined in severity, but her symptoms of tightness upon breathing, hacking cough, and profuse but difficult-to-expectorate sputum did not significantly improve. She came to our clinic.

INTAKE EXAMINATION
DATE: July 22, 1990

Her temperature was 37.8°C and she had a stifling sensation in her chest, tight breathing, a hacking cough, and sounds of sputum in her throat. The sputum was thick, jelly-like, profuse and frequently expectorated. After expectoration, the sputum was immediately replaced with a new supply. The patient was thirsty with a desire for cool liquids. Her tongue was red, lacked moisture, and had a thick, yellow, greasy coating. Her pulse was slippery and rapid and disappeared when strong pressure was applied.

DIFFERENTIATION OF PATTERNS AND DISCUSSION OF TREATMENT

DR. YU   Among phlegm diseases of the Lung system, it is relatively common to see a pattern of both phlegm-heat clogging the Lung and Lung dryness with damaged fluids. While this is case of a Lung infection occurring after an abdominal surgical procedure, it is like diseases such as acute bronchitis, bronchial asthma, lobar pneumonia, and exudative pleurisy in that at a certain stage of pathological change, a pattern of phlegm-heat clogging the Lung and Lung dryness with damaged fluids may develop.

The main symptoms of this pattern are a stifling sensation in the chest with wheezing, turbid, thick, sticky sputum that cannot be completely coughed up or spit out, and a dry mouth with a desire to drink, but with the act of drinking begetting a continuous hacking cough. If a large amount of the thick, sticky sputum rises to clog the throat it can lead to the acutely dangerous condition of respiratory arrest.

To effectively treat this kind of disorder it is necessary to use Phlegm-Dislodging Pill *(huò tán wán)*. According to Jiang Er-Xun's experience, other formulas or herbs are of no avail.

This was a pattern of phlegm-heat clogging the Lung and Lung dryness with damaged fluids. The treatment principle was to clear heat, dislodge phlegm, moisten what is dry and generate fluids.

To accomplish this, we prescribed a decoction of the herbs in Phlegm-Dislodging Pill *(huò tán wán)* from Tang Zong-Hai's *Discussion of Blood Patterns (Xuè zhèng lùn)*:

Angelicae sinensis Radix *(dāng guī)* 10g
Anemarrhenae Rhizoma *(zhī mǔ)* 10g
Trichosanthis Radix *(tiān huā fěn)* 15g
Cynanchi stauntonii Rhizoma *(bái qián)* 10g
Ophiopogonis Radix *(mài mén dōng)* 15g
Aurantii Fructus *(zhǐ ké)* 10g
Armeniacae Semen *(xìng rén)* 10g
Trichosanthis Semen *(guā lóu rén)* 12g
Platycodi Radix *(jié gěng)* 10g
Belamcandae Rhizoma *(shè gān)* 6g

Poria *(fú líng)* 15g
Dendrobii Herba *(shí hú)* 15g
untreated Glycyrrhizae Radix *(shēng gān cǎo)* 6g
fresh Bambusae Succus *(xiān zhú lì)*
   [divided into 3 doses and taken with strained decoction] 300ml

Instructions: Three packets were prescribed.

SECOND VISIT: After taking one packet the patient reported a significant reduction in the amount of thick, sticky sputum in her throat. When the three packets were finished, the patient no longer had phlegm-induced throat sounds, and there was a clear reduction in the intensity of the stifling sensation she felt in her chest and in her experience of wheezing and hacking cough. Her body temperature had also returned to normal. The only remaining symptoms were occasional coughing with expectoration of a small amount of sticky sputum, dull pain in the chest and lateral costal regions, a reddish tongue with a thin, yellow coating, and a pulse that was slightly rapid and that disappeared with strong pressure.

Remnants of phlegm-heat remained and there was discordance in the collaterals of the Lung. Thus, it was appropriate to clear heat, transform phlegm, clarify the Lung, and harmonize the collaterals.

For this we used an augmented version of Reed Decoction *(wěi jīng tāng)* from *Priceless and Important Formulas for Emergencies (Qiān jīn yào fāng)*:

untreated Coicis Semen *(shēng yì yǐ rén)* 20g
Benincasae Semen *(dōng guā zǐ)* 20g
Phragmitis Rhizoma *(lú gēn)* 30g
Persicae Semen *(táo rén)* 5g
Glehniae Radix *(běi shā shēn)* 15g
Armeniacae Semen *(xìng rén)* 10g
Curcumae Radix *(yù jīn)* 10g
Luffae Fructus Retinervus *(sī guā luò)* 15g

After taking five packets of this formula most of her symptoms dissipated. All that remained was a relative lack of energy, spirit, strength, and appetite. She was given a combination of Harmonize the Six Decoction *(liù hé tāng)* and Glehnia and Ophiopogonis Decoction *(shā shēn mài mén dōng tāng)* as a recuperative formula.

Disease	Primary symptoms	Differential diagnosis	Treatment method	Formula
Pneumonia with coughing & wheezing	cough, tight chest, thick & sticky sputum that returned immediately after expectoration	Phlegm-heat clogging the Lung, Lung dryness with damaged fluids	Clear heat, dislodge phlegm, moisten dryness, generate fluids	Phlegm-Dislodging Pill *(huò tán wán)*

REFLECTIONS AND CLARIFICATIONS

PHYSICIAN A   I have treated this type of situation using the traditional heat-clearing, phlegm-transforming formulas and herbs such as Clear the Qi and Transform Phlegm Pill *(qīng qì huà tán wán)*, *Minor Decoction [for Pathogens] Stuck in the Chest (xiǎo xiàn xiōng tāng)*, or, when severe, Flushing Away Roiling Phlegm Pill *(gǔn tán wán)*.

The results have been less than optimal.

Dr. Jiang initiated the use of Phlegm-Dislodging Pill *(huò tán wán)* and it achieves outstanding results. I recognize that this is a trail-blazing effort. However, this formula is rather complicated and difficult to understand.

DR. YU Dr. Jiang thought that to help patients with phlegm-heat clogging the Lung and Lung dryness with damaged fluids it is necessary to combine heat-clearing and phlegm-dislodging ingredients with those that moisten dryness and generate fluids. Only if the combination of ingredients precisely matches the condition will outstanding results be achieved.

However, agents that are commonly used to clear heat and transform phlegm not only lack any ability to moisten dryness and generate fluids, but because they are mostly bitter, cold substances that drain heat, consume qi and damage fluids, such as Coptidis Rhizoma *(huáng lián)*, Scutellariae Radix *(huáng qín)*, and Rhei Radix et Rhizoma *(dà huáng)*, they in fact exacerbate dryness.

Phlegm-Dislodging Pill *(huò tán wán)* can clear heat and dislodge phlegm without damaging the fluids, and can moisten dryness without causing phlegm to stagnate. While the formula's composition appears complex, it is actually quite straightforward.

- Platycodi Radix *(jié gěng)*, Glycyrrhizae Radix *(gān cǎo)*, Belamcandae Rhizoma *(shè gān)*, Poria *(fú líng)*, and Cynanchi stauntonii Rhizoma *(bái qián)* dispel phlegm, clear heat, disperse knots and improve the condition of the throat.

- Angelicae sinensis Radix *(dāng guī)*, Armeniacae Semen *(xìng rén)*, and Aurantii Fructus *(zhǐ ké)* stop coughing, settle wheezing, expand the chest and open the diaphragm.

- Anemarrhenae Rhizoma *(zhī mǔ)*, Trichosanthis Radix *(tiān huā fěn)*, Trichosanthis Fructus *(guā lóu)*, Ophiopogonis Radix *(mài mén dōng)*, and Dendrobii Herba *(shí hú)* enrich the Lung, moisten dryness, nourish the yin, and generate fluids.

- The most marvelous aspect of this approach is the use of fresh Bambusae Succus *(xiān zhú lì)* to flush out phlegm-heat from its lair and open areas clogged by phlegm-turbidity. Its effects are focused and its efficacy is impressive.

PHYSICIAN B When encountering phlegm-heat clogging the Lung and Lung dryness with damaged fluids one should avoid using sweet, warming substances as well as bland substances to leach out fluids. However, Phlegm-Dislodging Pill *(huò tán wán)* contains both sweet and warming Angelicae sinensis Radix *(dāng guī)* and blandly leaching Poria *(fú líng)*. This is also not easy to understand.

DR. YU It is said in the *Divine Husbandman's Classic of the Materia Medica (Shén Nóng běn cǎo jīng)* that Angelicae sinensis Radix *(dāng guī)* "governs cough and counterflow ascent of qi." Therefore it can stop coughing and calm wheezing. Most physicians have overlooked this. Simply because Angelicae sinensis Radix *(dāng guī)* is bitter and warm, does this mean that it is absolutely contraindicated in a pattern with symptoms of heat or yin damage? Not necessarily.

For example, tuberculosis is caused by a tuberculosis bacilli infection leading to erosion of lung tissue and a pattern of exhausted and injured Lung yin. This is why Zhu Dan-Xi explained that "consumption is primarily yin deficiency." Even up to the present time there is a widespread folk remedy for cough from pulmonary tuberculosis in which the main ingredient is Angelicae sinensis Radix *(dāng guī)*. In *Essentials of the Materia Medica (Běn cǎo bèi yào)* it is said that Angelicae sinensis Radix *(dāng guī)* "moistens dryness and lubricates the bowels"; thus, although it is warm, when paired with a large group of herbs that enrich the yin and moisten dryness, you can "ignore the nature and select by usefulness" to increase the herb combination's ability to moisten dryness and lubricate the bowels. The Lung and Large Intestine have an interior/exterior relationship, so when the bowels are lubricated and function smoothly it assists the clarifying and downward-directing functions of the Lung. I think this might be the reason that Angelicae sinensis Radix *(dāng guī)* has the functions of alleviating cough and calming wheezing.

As for Poria *(fú líng)*, *Essentials of the Materia Medica (Běn cǎo bèi yào)* states that it is "white in color and [consequently] enters the Lung, [where it] drains heat and unblocks the bladder, drains knotted pain in the epigastrium, [treats] chills and fever with irritability and fullness, parched mouth and dry tongue, coughing, retching, phlegm-fluids in the diaphragm … [it] generates fluids and relieves thirst." Herbs that enrich yin and moisten dryness are cloying and thus obstruct movement. Employing Poria *(fú líng)*, when using a large group of these sticky herbs, can prevent the obstruction of movement that is the shortcoming of their cloying nature.

PHYSICIAN B   You stated that this pattern can lead to an acutely dangerous condition when a large amount of the thick, sticky sputum flushes upward and obstructs the throat, leading to respiratory arrest. Can this formula be used in these critical situations?

DR. YU   Dr. Jiang used this formula to treat numerous patients with life-threatening conditions and got uniformly swift results. For example, on April 1, 1976 he saw a 30-year-old female patient on the Western medical wards. The patient was diagnosed with post-cholecystectomy syndrome (obstructive cholangitis) and toxic shock. Despite antibiotic and supportive treatments, her condition continued to worsen, and she also developed pneumonia with cough, profuse sputum, a stifling sensation in the chest, and rapid, shallow breathing. On the evening of March 23rd she suddenly stopped breathing due to a large amount of sputum that blocked her throat. An emergency tracheotomy was done under local anesthesia to clear out the sputum and prevent her from dying. However, large amounts of thick, sticky sputum came out of the opening, which required constant suction. She continued to require intravenous fluids and antibiotics. Things continued like this for the next seven days, her fever remaining high, and she went in and out of a semi-comatose condition.

When Dr. Jiang went to see the patient, she was listless and sleepy, she still had a large amount of sticky sputum coming from the tracheotomy, and she suffered from frequent gagging coughs and tight breathing. She was unable to swallow a food as simple as soup and was sweating profusely. Her tongue was red with a yellow, greasy coating and her pulse was slippery and rapid and lacked strength. He gave her Phlegm-Dislodging Pill *(huò tán wán)* with Generate the Pulse Powder *(shēng mài sǎn)*, including a large dosage of Bambusae Succus *(zhú lì)*. After taking one packet, the turbid sputum greatly decreased, she was able to take in a small amount of liquids, and the suction was successfully removed. Modified versions of the same formula were given for another 18 packets, after which the turbid sputum was almost completely eliminated, the patient recovered completely, and was discharged.

PHYSICIAN D   The original Phlegm-Dislodging Pill *(huò tán wán)* in *Discussion of Blood Patterns (Xuè zhèng lùn)* only has 3 *qián* [around 9g] of Bambusae Succus *(zhú lì)*, but in Dr. Jiang's formula the dosage is 300ml. Is it necessary to use such a large amount?

DR. YU   With Bambusae Succus *(zhú lì)* it is indeed necessary to use a large dosage! This is Dr. Jiang's experience in the clinic and also from his personal experience. Forty years ago, he had a chronic illness from phlegm and thin mucus. In the beginning he coughed, had chest and rib pain, and alternating malaria-like fevers and chills. He took Cyperus and Inula Decoction *(xiāng fù xuán fù huā tāng)* and recovered. Not long afterwards he caught another cold. There were no obvious signs of an external pattern, but he had a cough with copious sputum and a tight, pulling pain in his chest. He used Six-Serenity Decoction *(liù ān jiān)* to no effect, and then changed to Cyperus and Inula Decoction *(xiāng fù xuán fù huā tāng)*, which was also ineffective. He changed his physician many times, but none could make definitive progress.

The disease progressively worsened to the extent that simply breathing or twisting elicited the tight, pulling pain in his chest. All he could do was lay in bed, as he didn't dare move at all. He wheezed with a loud, phlegmy sound, his sputum was turbid, thick, and sticky with a stringy, molasses-like texture. He could force it up into his mouth but couldn't get it out except by scooping it out with his fingers. For seven days he couldn't eat or drink, and while his mouth was dry and he wanted to drink, when he took in water he would choke. He was on the verge of becoming critically ill.

His teacher, Chen Ding-San, told him to try Phlegm-Dislodging Pill *(huò tán wán)*. Because this was in the middle of the night, they didn't have access to Bambusae Succus *(zhú lì)* and so substituted turnip juice. After two packets, his condition had neither improved nor worsened and even his teacher felt helpless.

Just then someone came from the out of town asking Dr. Chen to come for a consultation, so he rushed off. At daybreak, Dr. Jiang's fellow students came to take a look at him, burning with concern. They set out numerous formulas, but Dr. Jiang shook them all off saying, "This is a Phlegm-Dislodging Pill *(huò tán wán)* presentation. On no account should we change the script."

He then urged someone to hurry and cut some bamboo and prepare a large amount of Bambusae Succus *(zhú lì)*, while Phlegm-Dislodging Pill *(huò tán wán)* was prepared as a decoction to which three cups (about 500ml) of the Bambusae Succus *(zhú lì)* would be added. He took the first dose at 3pm and the second dose at dusk. By the middle of the night he felt that the volume of turbid sputum was already decreasing and his wheezing and chest pain had also declined in severity. Unexpectedly, he was able to turn over. He took three more doses and by the next morning his symptoms had decreased significantly. The turbid sputum had not yet been spit up or drained downward, so he didn't know how it gradually ended up disappearing, but he did know that he was hungry and just wanted to eat.

After taking one more packet of the same formula, Dr. Jiang could walk around a bit if he used the bed as a support. Two days later he was able to go out. He then changed to using a formula to tonify both the qi and yin to recuperate for half of a month. His health then returned to the state it was in before he had fallen ill.

The personal nature of this experience of encroaching and then departing from the cusp of life and death was, as Dr. Jiang used to say, expressed in the saying, "Like a fish drinking water, one knows if it is cold or warm."

From this point forward, whenever Dr. Jiang used this formula to treat critical conditions owing to phlegm-heat clogging the Lung and Lung dryness with damaged fluids, he prescribed for the patient as he would have prescribed for himself and used a large amount of Bambusae Succus *(zhú lì)*. In the many times he employed this method, it never disappointed him.

Why does Bambusae Succus *(zhú lì)* have this outstanding effect? *Extension of the Materia Medica (Běn cǎo yǎn yì)* explains:

> Bambusae Succus *(zhú lì)* moves phlegm, from top to bottom, throughout the entire body from the hundred bones to the pores. Phlegm at the vertex is directed downward, while phlegm between the skin and the membranes can be moved. Also, epilepsy and mania, or spasms from wind-heat can be settled; those with aphasia or stupor from phlegm inversion can be brought back to awareness. This is a sage-like prescription for those suffering from phlegm.
>
> Clinical practice has proven that when large dosages of Bambusae Succus *(zhú lì)* are used, both its ability to clear heat and dislodge phlegm are magnified; it is without equal.

Based on Dr. Jiang's experience, the dosage of this substance for each dose of herbs should not be less than 60ml. While the original formulation of Phlegm-Dislodging Pill *(huò tán wán)* calls for bushy Bambusae Succus *(jīng zhú lì)*, Dr. Jiang would just use whatever bamboo grew locally, such as *dan zhu li* (Phyllostaehysnigra [Lodd.] Munro var. henonis [Mitf] Stapf ex Rendle), *ku zhu li* (Pleioblastus amarus), and *ci zhu li* (Neosinocalamus affinis[Rendli] Keng or Sinocalmus affinis [Rendle] McClure). While all of these have a reliable effect, bitter Bambusae Succus *(kǔ zhú lì)*, made from Pleioblastus amarus, is the best.

In summary, I would like to emphasize one more time that the key to achieving success with Phlegm-Dislodging Pill *(huò tán wán)* is to use a large dosage of Bambusae Succus *(zhú lì)*.

PHYSICIAN E   Dr. Yu, how is fresh Bambusae Succus *(zhú lì)* made?

DR. YU   The traditional method is as follows:

Cut fresh bamboo into sections delineated by the plant's growth sections. Cut off the joints at both ends of the section. Heat the middle of the section over a moderate flame and collect the liquid that is exuded from the two ends of the section.

PHYSICIAN E   Since fresh bamboo is not always available, can Bambusae Concretio silicea *(tiān zhú huáng)* be used as a substitute?

DR. YU Bambusae Concretio silicea *(tiān zhú huáng)* and Bambusae Succus *(zhú lì)* are both derived from bamboo. The *Comprehensive Outline of the Materia Medica (Běn cǎo gāng mù)* says that "The qi, flavor, and functions of Bambusae Concretio silicea *(tiān zhú huáng)* are the same as Bambusae Succus *(zhú lì)*, [but] Bambusae Concretio silicea *(tiān zhú huáng)* does not have the disadvantage that Bambusae Succus *(zhú lì)* has of being cold and slippery." While only a large dosage of Bambusae Succus *(zhú lì)* has the special function of flushing away phlegm-heat and opening obstruction from phlegm and oral mucus, Bambusae Concretio silicea *(tiān zhú huáng)* is more moderate and less apt to cause damage. Thus, Bambusae Concretio silicea *(tiān zhú huáng)* should be used as a substitute for Bambusae Succus *(zhú lì)*. To treat phlegm-heat clogging the Lung and Lung dryness with damaged fluids, use a large dosage of at least 15g as opposed to the normal dose of 3-6g. As the saying goes, "Even a clever daughter-in-law finds it difficult to cook without rice." What have we got to lose in trying Bambusae Concretio silicea *(tiān zhú huáng)* if no Bambusae Succus *(zhú lì)* is available? Also, I imagine that the natural version of Bambusae Concretio silicea *(tiān zhú huáng)* would be more like Bambusae Succus *(zhú lì)* than the synthetic substance often found in the herb markets nowadays.

CHAPTER 2

Generalized Disorders

2.1 Fever from internal damage

Six months of hot flushing, profuse sweating, and pain in the head and body

A confused state precedes a "trial treatment"

茫無頭緒先 "試探"

■ CASE HISTORY

Patient: *58-year-old female*

Half a year prior to our examination the patient had an injection of penicillin because of a urinary tract infection. Three days later a host of symptoms arose as an atypical allergic reaction: headache, red face, throat obstruction, numb hands and feet, generalized aches and pains, hot flushing, and profuse sweating.

After using both Chinese and Western medicines the symptoms declined markedly. Only the headaches, body pains, hot flushing, and profuse sweating remained unchanged. Despite undergoing a host of Western medical tests, no infection or other problem was discovered.

The patient's chart revealed that most of the herb formulas that she had taken had the functions of clearing heat, draining fire and enriching the yin, while simultaneously anchoring the yang. Intermixed among these were some formulas that aimed to expel wind and transform phlegm or dispel stasis and unblock the collaterals.

Intake Examination
Date: February 1, 1993

Every day in the early morning about two hours before dawn she develops a severe headache, with a burning forehead, generalized flushing, aches, dripping sweat, vomiting, and a fever of 37.5–38.5°C [99.5–103°F]. Despite taking pain pills when this occurs, she still moans and groans until dawn, by which time most of the symptoms have gradually resolved. Generalized aches, soreness and dizziness remain. During the day she is averse to cold and sweats when exposed to a draft. Her stools are slightly loose, and though her mouth is dry, she has no desire to drink. Her tongue body is red with a yellow, greasy coating and her pulse is sunken.

Differentiation of Patterns and Discussion of Treatment

PHYSICIAN A   When treating illness, Chinese medicine strives to "seek for the cause by assessing the pattern and determine the treatment by assessing the cause." In this case of six months of headache, body pain, hot flushing with profuse sweating, the clinical symptoms are complex and diverse, and the pulse and tongue seem to contradict the symptoms. Interior/exterior, heat/cold, excess/deficiency all are mixed up together and thus are hard to clearly differentiate. It is difficult even to grasp what exactly the chief complaint is and so the there is no firm ground upon which to establish a treatment plan. Therefore, all the treatments over this long period of time have been ineffective.

DR. YU   Not only is the course of this disease prolonged, the subjective symptoms are also complex and diverse, and Western medicine is unable to find any kind of focus of infection. Further, the tongue body is red with a yellow, greasy coating; this yellow and greasy coating seems out of place in the overall presentation. Parenthetically, if you pay attention to the medical adage that "in seasonal [externally-contracted] diseases, emphasize the pulse; in miscellaneous internal diseases, emphasize the tongue" you will fall into an overly rigid way of thinking. In Chapter 5 of the *Basic Questions (Sù wèn)* it states, "Those who excel at diagnosis inspect the complexion and take the pulse, first distinguishing yin and yang." In the end, is this a yin presentation or a yang presentation? I was at a loss and uncertain what to do.

After finishing the intake I sat and thought for a long time, as there is no way to prescribe a formula without grasping the main points of the problem. As you stated, interior/exterior, heat/cold, and excess/deficiency were all jumbled together and hard to clearly differentiate. I had no alternative but to use the "trial treatment" advocated by Zhang Zhong-Jing.[1]

Trial treatments require the use of formulas that serve as a trial test. This cannot be

....
1. *Translators' note:* This refers to line 209 of the *Discussion of Cold Damage (Shāng hán lùn)* where Minor Order the Qi Decoction *(xiǎo chéng qì tāng)* is recommended as a test to see whether someone who has not had a bowel movement for six or seven days should be purged. A sense of shifting of the full feeling in the abdomen and the passage of gas are evidence of the presence of dried feces; real purgatives, such as Major Order the Qi Decoction *(dà chéng qì tāng)*, are then recommended.

done without proper consideration. My experience has taught me that, for prolonged diseases that have not responded to numerous therapies, that have symptoms that are difficult to understand, and for which both the location and nature of the pathology are hard to determine, it is best to first try trial treatments using Bupleurum formulas such as Bupleurum and Cinnamon Twig Decoction (*chái hú guì zhī tāng*).

PHYSICIAN B   Why do you like trying Bupleurum and Cinnamon Twig Decoction (*chái hú guì zhī tāng*) in this case? Line 146 of the *Discussion of Cold Damage (Shāng hán lùn)* states, "Fever, slight chills, achy and uncomfortable joints of the limbs, slight retching, and propping knots below the heart [means] that the external pattern has not yet gone: Bupleurum and Cinnamon Twig Decoction (*chái hú guì zhī tāng*) governs it." This comes about from lack of resolution of an exterior *tài yáng* pathogen which then spreads to the *shào yáng* and so this formula is used. It is half Cinnamon Twig Decoction (*guì zhī tāng*), which releases the not completely spent *tài yáng* pathogen, and half Minor Bupleurum Decoction (*xiǎo chái hú tāng*), to resolve the slight knotting of the *shào yáng* condition.

This patient's condition has already lasted six months and so she not only lacks any incompletely released *tài yáng* pathogen, but also doesn't have slight *shào yáng* knotting. Why would you dispatch this formula as the spearhead to treat this patient?

DR. YU   Why would the relatively long duration of a disease preclude the existence of a Bupleurum (*chái hú*) presentation? As a younger person, Dr. Jiang once saw a woman who had been traumatized with fright from a fire and repeatedly exposed to cold. This led to her having alternating chills and fever for more than half a year. As the course of the disease had been prolonged, her constitution weakened and she became very sensitive to sounds; all the doctors who saw her treated her for deficient presentations. Dr. Jiang cured her with one packet of the original formulation of Minor Bupleurum Decoction (*xiǎo chái hú tāng*).

As the current case does display a Bupleurum (*chái hú*) presentation, I would not dream of casually dispensing Bupleurum and Cinnamon Twig Decoction (*chái hú guì zhī tāng*) and hoping for the best. So, why would I want to use this formula here? You all know that the scope of the *shào yáng* is very wide. As the Qing physician Chen Xiu-Yuan stated, "Externally, the *shào yáng* controls the interstices and pores; internally, it controls the Triple Burner." In this way, all the interstices and pores on the outside of a person's body, as well as the thoracic and abdominal cavities on the inside of the body, can be deemed as within the scope of *shào yáng*. Therefore, whenever I see a patient with a prolonged disorder that has failed multiple treatments, and where it is difficult to conclusively determine the site and nature of the disease due to a confusing set of signs and symptoms, I consider first using a Bupleurum (*chái hú*) prescription as a trial formula.

PHYSICIAN C   How do you choose a "trial treatment" and then progress towards a diagnosis? Isn't this a frustrating process of trial and error? We are especially interested in learning about this.

DR. YU   This process can certainly be described as one of trial and error.

Treatment and Outcome

First visit: One package of an augmented version of Bupleurum and Cinnamon Twig Decoction (chái hú guì zhī tāng) was given:

Bupleuri Radix (chái hú)..25g
Scutellariae Radix (huáng qín)..10g
standard Pinelliae Rhizoma praeparatum (fǎ bàn xià).....................10g
Codonopsis Radix (dǎng shēn)...15g
Glycyrrhizae Radix (gān cǎo)...5g
Cinnamomi Ramulus (guì zhī)..10g
Paeoniae Radix alba (bái sháo)..12g
Jujubae Fructus (dà zǎo) 15g
Zingiberis Rhizoma recens (shēng jiāng)..................................10g
Puerariae Radix (gé gēn) 30g
wine-fried Chuanxiong Rhizoma (jiǔ chǎo chuān xiōng) 30g
Pheretima (dì lóng) 10g

Second visit: Taking the formula had no effect. During the day the patient was averse to cold and was sweating more than before she took the formula; at night she experienced aches and pains in her head and body and increased tidal fevers. In addition, she had peri-orbital pain, pain in her chest and lateral costal regions, perianal burning, and semi-liquid stools. The tongue, pulse, and body temperature remained unchanged.

What does this demonstrate? On this day, after the patient had tried a dose of an augmented Bupleurum and Cinnamon Twig Decoction (chái hú guì zhī tāng), she absorbed the acrid, dispersing effects of such herbs as Bupleuri Radix (chái hú), Cinnamomi Ramulus (guì zhī), and wine-fried Chuanxiong Rhizoma (jiǔ chǎo chuān xiōng). This led to an increase in her diurnal sweating and aversion to cold, and resulted in no change to her pulse or tongue. This is the initial clue on the way toward determining that this was a yin-cold pattern. As such, the next step is to give one packet of Evodia Decoction (wú zhū yú tāng) as a trial treatment:

Evodiae Fructus (wú zhū yú)...15g
Codonopsis Radix (dǎng shēn)...20g
Jujubae Fructus (dà zǎo) 15g
Zingiberis Rhizoma recens (shēng jiāng)..................................20g

Third visit: The patient's diurnal aversion to cold and sweating decreased slightly, while the starting time of her head and body aches along with the tidal fevers and profuse sweating receded until 6-7 o'clock in the morning. Her nausea and vomiting decreased markedly and her temperature fell to 37.2°C [99°F].

With the use of the acrid, hot, purely yang Evodia Decoction (wú zhū yú tāng), all the symptoms were mitigated. This completely exposes the underlying foundation of a yin-cold pattern.

In the presence of a yang-heat pattern this trial treatment would have produced an entirely different patient condition. At this point the underlying pathodynamic of the condition was crystal clear: deficient and debilitated Kidney yang with cold congealing in the Liver and Stomach forcing yang qi to float upward and toward the exterior. With this in mind, one can confidently use a combination of:

- Aconite Accessory Root Decoction *(fù zǐ tāng)*
- Evodia Decoction *(wú zhū yú tāng)*
- Cinnamon Twig Decoction *(guì zhī tāng)*
- Jade Windscreen Powder *(yù píng fēng sǎn)*

Aconiti Radix lateralis praeparata *(zhì fù zǐ)* .... [precook for 30 minutes] 30g
Atractylodis macrocephalae Rhizoma *(bái zhú)* 20g
Paeoniae Radix alba *(bái sháo)* 15g
Poria *(fú líng)* 15g
Codonopsis Radix *(dǎng shēn)* 20g
Glycyrrhizae Radix praeparata *(zhì gān cǎo)* 6g
Evodiae Fructus *(wú zhū yú)* 15g
Jujubae Fructus *(dà zǎo)* 15g
Zingiberis Rhizoma recens *(shēng jiāng)* 20g
Cinnamomi Ramulus *(guì zhī)* 15g
Astragali Radix *(huáng qí)* 30g
Saposhnikoviae Radix *(fáng fēng)* 10g

Instructions: Three packets were given.

OUTCOME: After she finished the three packets of herbs, the patient's headaches, body pain, and tidal fevers and profuse sweating had ceased. Her aversion to cold and excess sweating during the day were significantly reduced, her temperature returned to normal, and her stools were now fully formed. Her tongue body was pale red with a thin, yellow, and slightly greasy coating, and her pulse was sunken.

She was given both Aconite Accessory Root Pill to Regulate the Middle *(fù zǐ lǐ zhōng wán)* and Tonify the Middle to Augment the Qi Decoction *(bǔ zhōng yì qì tāng)* in the form of pills to take for a month. By the end of the month her health had returned to normal.

PHYSICIAN A   That is fantastic! This "trial treatment" as advocated by Zhang Zhong-Jing is extraordinarily effective and helped you quickly discern which aspects of the presentation were red herrings and to eliminate the background noise in order to properly grasp the main symptoms and reveal the fundamental pathodynamic—deficient and debilitated Kidney yang with cold congealing in the Liver and Stomach forcing the yang qi to float upward and to the exterior.

However, for me, after using Evodia Decoction *(wú zhū yú tāng)* to reveal the yin-cold nature of this problem, it would be quite difficult to make the jump to such a finely crafted formula, as was used next.

DR. YU   It isn't difficult. Once the disease is clearly revealed to have a yin-cold nature, it would be hard for its location and degree of seriousness to suddenly change. At the same time, the proper treatment principle and composition of the formula flow naturally from an understanding of the underlying pattern.

For example, the patient's aversion to cold and sweating during the day along with nocturnal body aches and pains, watery stools, and sunken pulse can be presumed to be deficient and debilitated Kidney yang. As it says in line 305 of the *Discussion of*

Cold Damage (Shāng hán lùn), "For a *shào yīn* disease with body pain, cold hands and feet, and joint pain with a sunken pulse, Aconite Accessory Root Decoction *(fù zǐ tāng)* governs it."

As for the headache with retching and vomiting, this is Liver cold accosting the Stomach with counterflow ascent of turbid yin. Line 378 of the *Discussion of Cold Damage (Shāng hán lùn)* states, "For dry heaves, spitting up of mucus and froth, and headaches, Evodia Decoction *(wú zhū yú tāng)* governs it."

Regarding the symptoms of burning forehead, tidal fevers, and profuse sweating, these are signs of an internal overabundance of yin-cold forcing the yang qi to float upward and toward the exterior. For this reason, on a base of Aconite Accessory Root Decoction *(fù zǐ tāng)*, which warms and tonifies the Kidney yang, and Evodia Decoction *(wú zhū yú tāng)*, which warms the Liver and harmonizes the Stomach, we added Cinnamon Twig Decoction *(guì zhī tāng)* to transform qi and regulate yin and yang. The 17th-century author Xu Bin said of this formula, "For external patterns, it resolves the muscle layer and harmonizes the nutritive and protective qi; for internal patterns, it transforms qi and regulates yin and yang." Jade Windscreen Powder *(yù píng fēng sǎn)* was used to stabilize the exterior and stop sweating.

As you can see, isn't this a case where the strategy is established by the treatment principles and the formula emerges by following the strategy? Where is the difficulty?

Disease	Primary symptoms	Differential diagnosis	Treatment method	Formula
Fever from internal damage	Headache, body pains, flushing, profuse sweating	Deficient and debilitated Kidney yang; cold congealing in the Liver and Stomach	Warm the yang and disperse cold	Aconite Accessory Root Decoction *(fù zǐ tāng)*, Evodia Decoction *(wú zhū yú tāng)*

REFLECTIONS AND CLARIFICATIONS

PHYSICIAN B   The difficulty in differentiating the yin-cold presentation in this case is that the yin-cold symptoms are few and vague while the yang-heat symptoms are both numerous and prominent. In other words, the manifestations of yang-heat eclipse the yin-cold nature of the pattern. Nowadays, people consider this type of disease process to be 'fever from internal damage', and in the lineage of the Jin-Yuan physician Li Dong-Yuan it is called 'yin fire.'

PHYSICIAN C   The basic pathodynamic of what Li Dong-Yuan called 'yin fire' is Spleen deficiency with sinking qi; but in this case the main issue is deficient and debilitated Kidney yang. Recently, some notable physicians have taken presentations from the *Discussion of Cold Damage (Shāng hán lùn)*, such as those for Unblock the Pulse Decoction for Frigid Extremities *(tōng mài sì nì tāng)* and White Penetrating Decoction *(bái tōng tāng)*, characterized by deficient and debilitated Kidney yang with internal flourishing of yin-cold that barricades the yang upwards or toward the exterior, and classified them as 'Kidney deficiency yin-fire.' In this way they have continued and extended the work of Li Dong-Yuan.

Clinically, if you can employ this type of thinking, it enables you to very quickly penetrate the false signs of 'fire-heat' to clearly see the essential yin-cold quality beneath. This prevents one from succumbing to the predicament of "wandering among the symptoms without a set perspective." Do you agree?

DR. YU   I could not casually agree with this. As Confucius said, "If names are not correct, language will not be not in accordance with the truth; if language is not in accordance with the truth, affairs cannot be successfully carried out."

PHYSICIAN B   How does "If names are not correct, language will not be in accordance with the truth" relate to what we are discussing?

DR. YU   Fire cannot be divided into yin and yang.

PHYSICIAN B   Why can fire not be divided into yin and yang? Lao-zi said, "The myriad things have yin on their back and embrace yang." In Chapter 5 of the *Basic Questions (Sù wèn)* it states, "Yin and yang are the way of heaven and earth, the guiding principles of the myriad things." These sources see yin and yang as being the basic directive for the myriad things and the cosmos. Can it be that 'fire' is outside of the myriad things?

DR. YU   Answering this question involves a proper understanding of the philosophical scope of the 'yin-yang' pair. As you all know, while the yin-yang pairing possesses the universal attribute of the unity of opposites, at the same time it has some special qualitative aspects as it represents a special direction of motion and state of motion. Because of this, yin-yang does not have the same scope as the concept of 'contradiction' has in dialectical materialism, where it is the most ideal and generalized summary of all objects and phenomena in the natural world.

The contemporary philosopher Liu Chang-Lin (劉長林) observes in *The Philosophy of the Inner Classic and the Methodology of Chinese Medicine (Nèi jīng zhé xué hé zhōng yī xué de fāng fǎ)* that "Yin-yang has its own special qualitative aspects and belongs to one group of specific contradictions, so its scope of application must have certain limits, and cannot have unlimited applications. … Due to the limitations of direct observation, quite a few phenomena are difficult to place within the categories of yin and yang." This is to say that while the ancients subjectively desired to use the categories of yin and yang to explain everything, in reality, that cannot be done.

As there are definite limitations to specific usages of yin and yang, whether a given thing in the end can be differentiated into yin and yang requires a specific analysis of the specific question.

Now we are focused in this way on 'fire.' There is a wide variety of types of fire, but in general we can divide them into two broad categories, normal or upright fire, known as lesser fire (少火 *shào huǒ*), and pathogenic fire, known as vigorous fire (壯 火 *zhuàng huǒ*):

- Normal fire is the one aspect of the body's normal qi that has the quality of warming and generating. Chapter 5 of the *Basic Questions (Sū wèn)* says of it, "The lesser fire generates qi."

- Pathogenic qi (which includes internal fire, external fire, fire from deficiency, and fire from excess) pertains to pathological fire. It is generated by an overabundance of yang and is the epitome of heat. Its nature is to flare upwards and scorch. It damages and consumes fluids, generates wind, and stirs the blood. It is a purely yang pathogen, so how could it have even the least bit of yin qualities?

We can see from this that while there are many types of fire, there is no way to divide them into yin or yang. In the same way, there is no way to divide cold into 'yang cold' or 'yin cold.'

PHYSICIAN A You have written a few articles setting out your contentious views on 'yin fire.' Although these are just one person's words, they have a basis and there are grounds for this view. However, the concept of pathological 'yin fire' has been used for a long time and I'm afraid that it will continue to be used. This is because up to now, no better term has been developed to take its place for this pathological condition. If one doesn't use it, then it is rather troublesome to talk about this type of presentation. Doesn't it seem that way to you?

DR. YU There are famous doctors who never used the term 'yin fire' and still were able to speak convincingly and with authority. For example, the renowned early-modern physician Zhang Xi-Chun in his notes to the formula he created called Regulate Thin Mucus Decoction *(lǐ yǐn tāng)* [2] wrote about the pathological pattern for which it is indicated:

> This treats Heart and Lung yang deficiency that leads to the Spleen [being encumbered by] dampness and not directing upwards and the Stomach being constrained and not directing downwards, so that foodstuffs are unable to be transported and transformed into the essentials [of nutrition] and instead change to become pathogenic thin mucus. … When severe, this [thin mucus] may form a haze that blankets the entire upper burner so that yang qi of the Heart and Lung is unable to flow smoothly. This converts into constraint, which then produces heat. Alternatively, yin qi compels yang qi to travel to the exterior where it manifests as corporal fever or it may compel yang qi to float upwards and develop into deafness.

Both the medicine and the writing here are remarkable and reflect well upon each other. The description of the pathodynamic in this case is based, in part, on this thinking.

....

2. This is Poria, Cinnamon Twig, Atractylodes, and Licorice Decoction *(líng guì zhú gān tāng)* plus Paeoniae Radix alba *(bái sháo)*, Citri reticulatae Pericarpium *(chén pí)*, Zingiberis Rhizoma *(gān jiāng)*, and Magnoliae officinalis Cortex *(hòu pò)*.

CHAPTER 3

Gynecology and Obstectrics

3.1 Vaginal discharge

A case of a vaginal discharge for more than two years

Ancient formulas don't have much to do with modern diseases

古方今病不相能

■ CASE HISTORY

Patient: *35-year-old woman*

The patient reported excessive vaginal discharge for more than two years. The gynecology department diagnosed her with chronic pelvic inflammatory disease. Approximately two years ago, the patient underwent a dilatation and curettage following a failed attempt at a drug-induced abortion. Following this procedure, she developed an infection that led to acute pelvic inflammatory disease.

She was treated with large doses of antibiotics, which controlled the acute infection. However, the disease recurred and became chronic. For more than two years now she has had excessive vaginal discharge that is primarily yellow, with sometimes a white-yellow mix, and occasionally also displaying grayish-brown, green, or pink aspects. The discharge is thick and foul smelling.

Through vaginal smear, her physician ruled out yeast, trichomoniasis, and sexually-transmitted diseases. Courses of erythromycin, ampicillin, ofloxacin, and norfloxacin were helpful at first, but as soon as the medications were stopped, the symptoms returned.

From a Chinese medicine perspective, she was diagnosed with damp-heat in the lower burner and treated with modifications of a combination of Gentian Decoction to Drain the Liver *(lóng dǎn xiè gān tāng)* and Four-Marvel Powder *(sì miào sǎn)* for more than ten packets with poor results. Treatment with modifications of a combination of Change Yellow [Discharge] Decoction *(yì huáng tāng)* and Four-Marvel Powder *(sì miào sǎn)* were also ineffective.

INTAKE EXAMINATION
JULY 18, 1996

The patient's symptoms were as described above. Her complexion was dark and dull. She reported shortness of breath, weakness, lumbosacral pain, a tendency towards dry stool, and yellow, scanty urine. Her menstrual cycle was long with scanty black blood. During her menstrual flow, she suffered distention and pain in her lower abdomen. Her tongue was dusky and pale with a thin, yellow coating and her pulse was wiry and sunken.

DIFFERENTIATION OF PATTERNS AND DISCUSSION OF TREATMENT

PHYSICIAN A   Vaginal discharge occurs commonly and is frequently seen in gynecology clinics. In Western medicine, it is frequently considered a symptom of inflammation affecting the reproductive system and treatment commonly uses antibiotics. In this case of yellow vaginal discharge, the physician had ruled out gynecologic tumors, and the patient was diagnosed with chronic pelvic inflammatory disease, which was considered a damp-heat pattern. However, long-term treatment with antibiotics as well as herbal formulas to clear heat and resolve dampness was ineffective. Could it be that the traditional concept that "vaginal discharge pertains to dampness" is obsolete?

DR. YU   No, the concept that vaginal discharge belongs to dampness and that yellow discharge belongs to damp-heat is not obsolete. In *Fu Qing-Zhu Women's Disorders (Fù Qīng-Zhǔ nǚ kē)*, the 17th-century author Fu Qing-Zhu writes, "Vaginal discharge (带 下 *dài xià*) is a damp disease. The character 带 *(dài)* is used in the name of this disease because it is caused by a failure of the binding action of the Girdle *(dài)* vessel." This passage clearly expresses that the etiology of vaginal discharge combines dampness and a failure of the binding action of the Girdle vessel.

    In the same text, there is a discussion of yellow vaginal discharge which states that, "In women with vaginal discharge that is yellow, like concentrated tea that smells fishy and dirty, this is called yellow vaginal discharge. It is the result of damp-heat affecting the Conception vessel." Dr. Fu recommends the formula Change Yellow [Discharge] Decoction *(yì huáng tāng)*, which is composed of a large dosage (30g) of Dioscoreae Rhizoma *(shān yào)* and Euryales Semen *(qiàn shí)* to tonify the deficiency of the Conception vessel, ten pieces of Ginkgo Semen *(bái guǒ)* to restrain and stabilize the Girdle vessel, and small amounts of brine-fried Phellodendri Cortex *(huáng bǎi)* (6g) and wine-fried Plantaginis Semen *(chē qián zǐ)* (3g) to assist in clearing and draining damp-heat from the lower burner. Dr. Fu also describes the superior efficacy of the formula: "After continuously taking four packets, all cases will be cured. This formula is not only suitable for yellow discharge but can be used in all cases. However, it is an even more miraculous treatment for yellow discharge."

In the 1970s I tested this formula in the clinic for yellow vaginal discharge. Prescribing it by itself, I did not find it to be particularly effective. I then used it in combination with strong formulas that resolve dampness, clear heat, and resolve toxicity such as Gentian Decoction to Drain the Liver *(lóng dǎn xiè gān tāng)*, Four-Marvel Powder *(sì miào sǎn)*, and Five-Ingredient Drink to Eliminate Toxin *(wǔ wèi xiāo dú yǐn)* in order to fight hard against the momentum of the disease, and only after this found an effective combination by using Change Yellow [Discharge] Decoction *(yì huáng tāng)* with Discharge-clearing Decoction *(qīng dài tāng)* from Zhang Xi-Chun, which is composed of Dioscoreae Rhizoma *(shān yào)* 30g, Fossilia Ossis Mastodi *(lóng gǔ)* 18g, Ostreae Concha *(mǔ lì)* 18g, Sepiae Endoconcha *(hǎi piāo xiāo)* 12g, and Rubiae Radix *(qiàn cǎo gēn)* 6g.

PHYSICIAN B   Do you mean to say that Fu Qing-Zhu exaggerated his results and should not serve as a model for treatment?

DR. YU   No! Fu Qing-Zhu was a virtuous physician to whom contemporaries showed great respect, saying that "His medicine, excellent as it is, is inferior to his works of literature, which are inferior to his poetry, which is yet inferior to him as a person." Many of the formulas in *Fu Qing-Zhu Women's Disorders (Fù Qīng-Zhǔ nǚ kē)* have shown enduring clinical utility. If Change Yellow [Discharge] Decoction *(yì huáng tāng)* is an exception, there must be a reason.

  If we infer the pattern from the formula, we could conclude that Dr. Fu considered yellow vaginal discharge to be the result of a relatively severe deficiency of Spleen and Kidney, as well as the Conception and Girdle vessels, accompanied by relatively mild damp-heat in the lower burner. This pattern is 'more deficiency than excess' and 'more cold than heat.' In the case of the yellow vaginal discharge that we are discussing, however, the patient belongs to a pattern of mixed deficiency and excess combined with mixed heat and cold. Furthermore, the excess in this case involves pathogenic toxin and blood stasis, representing a case of "times change, generations shift, and ancient and modern paths diverge."

PHYSICIAN B   How did there come to be pathogenic toxin and blood stasis in this case?

DR. YU   Gynecologic procedures, such as placing an IUD, surgical abortion, medical abortion, labor induction, loop electrosurgical excision procedure, and laser treatments, as well as gynecologic medications, can directly injure the Womb as well as the Conception and Girdle vessels. Damp-heat pathogenic toxin can take advantage of this injury-induced deficiency to enter. The implements used in these procedures can directly damage the collateral vessels, causing excessive bleeding. Once the blood leaves the vessels, it can become static and lead to stasis-obstruction of the collateral vessels. The mixing of pathogenic toxin and blood stasis within damp-heat is an important factor in treatment-resistant vaginal discharge.

PHYSICIAN C   If I follow your thinking that "times change, generations shift, and ancient and modern paths diverge," is it fair to say that ancient formulas are incompatible with modern diseases?

DR. YU   At least in the case of damp-heat vaginal discharge, yes, it is possible to say that. If you treat damp-heat vaginal discharge using the standard methods without success over an extended period of time, you must advance one step further in assessing the patterns and seeking the cause. As it states in Chapter 74 of the Basic Questions *(Sū wèn)*, "Carefully monitor the disease dynamics and in each case manage what [signs and symptoms] are associated with it. When [signs and symptoms] are present, investigate them. When [signs and symptoms] are absent, investigate them." You must proceed to determine if there is concomitant pathogenic toxin and/or blood stasis.

The pattern differentiation for this case was deficiency of essence qi, and damp toxin combined with static heat piling up in the pelvic cavity.

I decided to tonify qi and boost essence, dispel dampness, resolve toxicity, transform stasis, and clear heat, but was concerned that in the near term, using tonics could possibly "block the door and retain the enemy." Thus, I started with a formula to dispel dampness, resolve toxicity, transform stasis, and clear heat.

TREATMENT AND OUTCOME

The formula was a combination of Pulsatilla Decoction *(bái tóu wēng tāng)* and Five-Ingredient Drink to Eliminate Toxin *(wǔ wèi xiāo dú yǐn)* with modifications:

Pulsatillae Radix *(bái tóu wēng)*	30g
Coptidis Rhizoma *(huáng lián)*	5g
scorched Phellodendri Cortex *(jiāo huáng bǎi)*	10g
Fraxini Cortex *(qín pí)*	15g
Taraxaci Herba *(pú gōng yīng)*	30g
Violae Herba *(zǐ huā dì dīng)*	30g
Lonicerae Flos *(jīn yín huā)*	15g
Chrysanthemi indici Flos *(yě jú huā)*	30g
Lycopi Herba *(zé lán)*	15g
Moutan Cortex *(mǔ dān pí)*	10g
Persicae Semen *(táo rén)*	10g

Instructions: Six packets were prescribed.

SECOND VISIT: All of the patient's symptoms remained unchanged except that her bowels and urination were smoother and easier than before.

I thought about this situation for a long time until I had an insight. I changed the formula to a combination of Pulsatilla Decoction *(bái tóu wēng tāng)* and Coix, Aconite Accessory Root, and Patrinia Powder *(yì yǐ fù zǐ bài jiàng sǎn)* with modifications:

Pulsatillae Radix *(bái tóu wēng)*	30g
Coptidis Rhizoma *(huáng lián)*	10g
scorched Phellodendri Cortex *(huáng bǎi)*	10g
Fraxini Cortex *(qín pí)*	15g
Coicis Semen *(yì yǐ rén)*	60g
Aconiti Radix lateralis praeparata *(zhì fù zǐ)*	10g
Patriniae Herba *(bài jiàng cǎo)*	30g
Cimicifugae Rhizoma *(shēng má)*	30g
Astragali Radix *(huáng qí)*	50g

Bruceae Fructus *(yā dǎn zǐ)* .... 30 pieces
    (each one is stuffed into a Longan Arillus *(lóng yǎn ròu)*—10 pieces
    each time—and washed down with the strained cooked decoction)[1]
powdered Notoginseng Radix *(sān qī)* .... [as a draft; 2g per dose] 6g

Instructions: Six packets were prescribed, three doses each day.

THIRD VISIT: The patient's yellow vaginal discharge had greatly decreased, her gray-ish-brown and pink discharges had ceased, and the shortness of breath and weakness she had been experiencing improved. However, the lumbosacral pain persisted and her tongue and pulse were largely unchanged. We then changed to Coix, Aconite Accessory Root, and Patrinia Powder *(yì yǐ fù zǐ bài jiàng sǎn)* combined with some elements of Reduced Formula to Calm Low Back Pain *(jiǎn wèi yào tòng níng)*, an experiential formula from a famous local doctor, Chen Si-Yi (陳思義):

Coicis Semen *(yì yǐ rén)* 60g
Aconiti Radix lateralis praeparata *(zhì fù zǐ)* 10g
Patriniae Herba *(bài jiàng cǎo)* 30g
Astragali Radix *(huáng qí)* 50g
Angelicae sinensis Radix *(dāng guī)* 15g
Taxilli Herba *(sāng jì shēng)* 15g
Dipsaci Radix *(xù duàn)* 15g
Eucommiae Cortex *(dù zhòng)* 15g
Psoraleae Fructus *(bǔ gǔ zhī)* 20g
Cuscutae Semen *(tù sī zǐ)* .... [wrapped] 30g
Smilacis glabrae Rhizoma *(tǔ fú líng)* 30g
powdered Notoginseng Radix *(sān qī)* .... [as a draft; 2g per dose] 6g

RESULT: After taking 24 packets of the preceding formula, the patient's yellow vaginal discharge ceased, her lumbosacral region felt good, and her dark and dull complexion had greatly improved. However, the tongue remained a dusky, pale color and it appeared that this pattern, in which stasis had congealed deeply within the collateral vessels, could not be resolved through the use of a decoction. We therefore changed to a powder in order to slowly transform stasis and unblock the collaterals, which is referred to as "using a powder (散 *sǎn*) to disperse (散 *sàn*)." I gave her powdered Notoginseng Radix *(sān qī)* 360g and had her take 2g, three times each day, as a draft. She continued this for two months to consolidate the treatment outcome.

Disease	Primary symptoms	Differential diagnosis	Treatment method	Formula
Vaginal discharge	Yellow, thick, and foul smelling vaginal discharge	Deficiency of essence qi, and damp toxin intermingled with static heat	Tonify qi and boost essence, dispel dampness, resolve toxicity, transform stasis, and clear heat	Pulsatilla Decoction *(bái tóu wēng tāng)* with Coix, Aconite Accessory Root, and Patrinia Powder *(yì yǐ fù zǐ bài jiàng sǎn)*

....

1. *Translators' note:* Bruceae Fructus *(yā dǎn zǐ)* is corrosive and thus needs the protection of the Longan Arillus *(lóng yǎn ròu)* to carry it safely into the stomach, not irritating the mouth, throat or esophagus.

REFLECTIONS AND CLARIFICATIONS

PHYSICIAN C   Why, in this case of vaginal discharge, did you begin treatment with Pulsatilla Decoction *(bái tóu wēng tāng)*, which is a formula for *jué yīn* dysentery?

DR. YU   Pulsatilla Decoction *(bái tóu wēng tāng)* is originally found in the *jué yīn* chapter of *Discussion of Cold Damage (Shāng hán lùn)* and there are two related lines from the source text. Line 371 reads, "For hot diarrhea with tenesmus, Pulsatilla Decoction *(bái tóu wēng tāng)* governs it." Line 373 reads, "Diarrhea with a desire to drink fluids is due to the presence of heat: Pulsatilla Decoction *(bái tóu wēng tāng)* governs it." I think that these can be attributed to damp-heat in the Liver channel disturbing the Large Intestine and damaging the collateral vessels, which causes tenesmus and diarrhea containing pus and blood. When Liver channel damp-heat pours into the pelvic cavity, it damages the Womb as well as the Conception, Girdle, and Penetrating vessels. This damage produces a similar response in the female reproductive system, which results in vaginal discharge containing pus and blood. As these are two branches diverging from one source, the treatments are similar.

The primary ingredient in the formula, Pulsatillae Radix *(bái tóu wēng)*, "drives out blood and stops dysentery," according to *Divine Husbandman's Classic of the Materia Medica (Shén Nóng běn cǎo jīng)*. Further, according to *Miscellaneous Records of Famous Physicians (Míng yī bié lù)*, it also "stops toxic diarrhea." Pulsatillae Radix *(bái tóu wēng)* clears the Liver and cools the blood; it transforms stasis and resolves toxicity. In this formula, it is combined with Coptidis Rhizoma *(huáng lián)* and Phellodendri Cortex *(huáng bǎi)* to clear heat, dry dampness, and resolve toxicity, as well as Fraxini Cortex *(qín pí)*, which, being green, enters the Liver and clears heat, fortifies yin, and stops vaginal discharge.

Although the formula matches the pattern, it has a relatively weak ability to resolve toxicity. Thus, we combined it with Five-Ingredient Drink to Eliminate Toxin *(wǔ wèi xiāo dú yǐn)*, from the *Golden Mirror of the Medical Tradition (Yī zōng jīn jiàn)*, to strengthen its ability to resolve toxicity and clear heat. However, the effect was still poor, indicating that the stasis and toxin were relatively severe. So I drew a lesson from a special method developed by the famous modern physician Zhang Xi-Chun in which he used Bruceae Fructus *(yā dǎn zǐ)* and powdered Notoginseng Radix *(sān qī)* to resolve toxicity and transform stasis. This approach is generally effective.

PHYSICIAN A   When the patient came in, you observed that perhaps there was an element of damp toxin and stasis, which you addressed through the formula you chose, but the condition did not improve and seemed to be quite persistent. What surprised me was that you made the decision to use Coix, Aconite Accessory Root, and Patrinia Powder *(yì yǐ fù zǐ bài jiàng sǎn)*, which is a formula from the *Essentials from the Golden Cabinet (Jīn guì yào lüè)* that treats an intestinal abscess with pus, and this approach was quickly effective. You have not yet explained your rationale for using this formula.

DR. YU   As you mentioned, Coix, Aconite Accessory Root, and Patrinia Powder *(yì yǐ fù zǐ bài jiàng sǎn)* is cited in Chapter 18 of *Essentials from the Golden Cabinet (Jīn* *guì yào lüè)*: "In the disease of intestinal abscess, the skin is scaly, and the abdominal skin is tense, yet soggy when pressed, as if it is swollen. Abdominal accumulations and clusters are absent, as is fever, and the pulse is rapid. This is a purulent abscess in the intestine and Coix, Aconite Accessory Root, and Patrinia Powder *(yì yǐ fù zǐ bài jiàng sǎn)* governs it." The large dosage of Coicis Semen *(yì yǐ rén)* opens clogged areas and expels pus. Patriniae Herba *(bài jiàng cǎo)* dissipates abscesses and expels pus and invigorates the blood and transforms stasis. Aconiti Radix lateralis praeparata *(zhì fù zǐ)*, used in a small dosage as an assistant, stimulates the yang and unblocks stasis through warmth. This formula is appropriate when pus has already formed in an intestinal abscess (which is equivalent to an appendicular abscess), and when the body's yang qi is insufficient and the normal qi cannot overcome the pathogen. In recent years, there have been clinical reports of using this formula in conjunction with antibiotics to cure abscessed appendix, without the need for surgery.

In the above example of using this formula for yellow vaginal discharge, I not only made use of the formula's ability to expel pus and dispel stasis, but also relied on the action of Aconiti Radix lateralis praeparata *(zhì fù zǐ)* to warm yang to increase movement through areas of stagnation.

PHYSICIAN A   And yet, in this case of yellow vaginal discharge, there were signs of neither yang deficiency nor cold stagnation, so why would you use Aconiti Radix lateralis praeparata *(zhì fù zǐ)* to warm yang and promote movement through stagnant areas?

DR. YU   When an area of stagnation is exposed to cold, it tends to worsen, whereas when exposed to heat, it warms up and thus there is proper movement through it. In patterns of damp-heat with toxin and stasis, it can be difficult to avoid unknowingly injuring the yang qi as a result of prolonged use of substances that clear heat, resolve dampness, and transform stasis in conjunction with antibiotics. (From the viewpoint of Chinese medicine, antibiotics are considered a cooling substance.)

In this case, the patient's complexion was dark and dull, she had shortness of breath, weakness, and lumbosacral pain. Her tongue was dusky and pale with a thin, yellow coating. Her pulse was wiry and sunken. Is this not evidence of yang deficiency and cold stagnation? It probably is. When yang is deficient, the functions of warming, warm unblocking, and warm dispersing all lack force. If left untreated, the momentum will move towards the next stage of damage to yang qi. Thus, we used 10g of Aconiti Radix lateralis praeparata *(zhì fù zǐ)* to warm and unblock the yang qi. In addition, I added a large dosage (50g) of Astragali Radix *(huáng qí)* to raise and tonify the great qi.

As Zhang Zhong-Jing noted in Chapter 14 of *Essentials from the Golden Cabinet (Jīn guì yào lüè)*, "As soon as the great qi shifts, the knotting will disperse." What does he mean by 'knotting'? In my opinion, knotting refers to aggravated clusters of pathogens such as phlegm-dampness, blood stasis, and pathogenic toxin taking shape within the body. Vaginal discharge belongs to this category.

PHYSICIAN B   I find many new ideas in what you have explained so far. However, in thinking about vaginal discharge, classical and modern physicians have primarily relied on the amount, color, quality, and smell to assist in classification and treatment. In modern Chinese medicine publications, we find four major classifications for vaginal discharge: Spleen deficiency, Kidney deficiency, damp-heat, and damp-toxin. Even in the case of red vaginal discharge, it is classified generally as yin deficiency with internal heat accompanied by dampness and is not attributed to blood stasis. In your discussion of vaginal discharge, in the case of not only red discharge but also white and yellow discharge, you place significant importance on determining the presence or absence of static blood. This idea is truly original.

DR. YU   In fact, this idea is not original, but was already present in the classics. In Chapter 22 on miscellaneous diseases in women in *Essentials from the Golden Cabinet (Jīn guì yào lüè)*, it states, "When menstrual flow is blocked and does not flow and there is hardness and intractable ensconced lumps in the Womb, it indicates dry blood inside; there will be a white substance [discharged]." The "white substance" mentioned in this line refers to vaginal discharge and the "dry blood" mentioned is another term for static blood. This line clearly indicates that the cause of white vaginal discharge is static blood. In *Correction of Errors Among Physicians (Yī lín gǎi cuò)*, Qing-dynasty physician Wang Qing-Ren discusses the treatment of lower abdominal accumulations and pain using Drive out Stasis from the Lower Abdomen Decoction *(shào fù zhú yū tāng)*. He also clearly states that this formula can treat white vaginal discharge, which demonstrates that this type of vaginal discharge can be the result of static blood.

In the early years of the Republican period in China, the famous physician Tang Zong-Hai also discussed white vaginal discharge. Although he stated that it was "primarily focused in the Spleen" and that one should "harmonize the Spleen to promote urination," he also pointed out that vaginal discharge is "the result of damage to the blood of the Girdle vessel." Isn't this damage to the blood related to static blood? Unfortunately, Dr. Tang did not tie this all together by offering a specific treatment method.

In thinking about cases of vaginal discharge in the modern clinic, I have a strong feeling of "the difference between the past and the present." In clinical practice, one must be careful not to superficially peruse textbooks or to write about clinical issues in clichés. What do I mean by this? The case above is a mixed pattern of deficiency and excess with more excess and less deficiency; a mixed pattern of cold and heat with more heat and less cold. Vaginal discharge owing to damp-heat is the most common pattern observed. When it is resistant to treatment, one must carefully consider the possibility that pathogenic toxin and/or static blood are harbored within the body. Furthermore, in the treatment of vaginal discharge from damp-heat with toxin and stasis, it is appropriate to use a foundation of substances that clear heat, resolve dampness, resolve toxicity and transform stasis. To this foundation, one should add a large dosage of Astragali Radix *(huáng qí)* to tonify qi and disperse knots while at the same time assisting with a small dosage of Aconiti Radix lateralis praeparata *(zhì fù zǐ)* and Cinnamomi Ramulus *(guì zhī)* to warm yang with the aim of increasing movement through areas of stagnation. In this way, one can achieve success.

3.2 Irregular uterine bleeding

Two cases of severe irregular uterine bleeding

Clinical efficacy comes easily with a specialized formula

高效专方一用就灵

■ CASE HISTORY 1

Patient No. 1: *Ms. Luo, 42-year-old female*

The patient presented with a six-month history of recurrent, irregular uterine bleeding. She had repeatedly used hormones and Chinese herbal medicines without any effect. Having undergone a diagnostic dilatation and curettage, she was diagnosed with luteal phase defect. The gynecology department recommended that she have a hysterectomy, but she feared the surgery and instead placed her hopes in Chinese herbal treatment.

INTAKE EXAMINATION
DATE: July 26, 1985

Ms. Luo experienced continuous light uterine bleeding punctuated by profuse, clot-containing bleeding every few days. Her complexion was very pale and she had deficiency-type superficial facial edema. She was weak and short of breath. Her tongue was pale and her pulse was wiry, fine, and rough.

■ CASE HISTORY 2

Patient No. 2: *Ms. You, 15-year-old female*

The patient reported a six-month history of continuous light uterine bleeding punctuated by frequent episodes of profuse bleeding. She experienced menarche at age 13 and soon after contracted 'myocarditis.' She frequently took Western medicine but was unable to regain her health completely and her constitution weakened. She was diagnosed with 'dysfunctional uterine bleeding' and had undergone three blood transfusions. She had used hemostatic and anti-inflammatory medications as well as hormones but the bleeding persisted. She had also tried more than 30 packets of Chinese herbs without effect. This herbal treatment included formulas to clear heat and cool the blood, invigorate the blood and transform stasis, tonify the qi and contain blood, and replenish and bind essence. She also tried home remedies and experiential formulas. The patient's mother was an attending gynecological physician at a hospital and she was at her wit's end about this situation. She was extremely anxious about her daughter's condition and ultimately made the decision to bring her to the Leshan Hospital to see the renowned physician, my teacher Jiang Er-Xun. When the patient arrived at the hospital, she was so weak that she had to be carried from the car into the exam room.

INTAKE EXAMINATION (by Jiang Er-Xun)
DATE: May 20, 1988

The patient had superficial edema over her entire body. Her complexion was pale, her voice low, and she was short of breath. When she moved, her breath became more rapid. Her lips and tongue were pale. With deep pressure, her pulses were imperceptible and with light pressure they were barely discernible.

DIFFERENTIATION OF PATTERNS AND DISCUSSION OF TREATMENT

DR. YU   In my early career I tried many formulas to treat severe irregular uterine bleeding with unsatisfactory results. I overcame this obstacle while reviewing *Essays on Medicine Esteeming the Chinese and Respecting the Western (Yī xué zhōng zhōng cān xī lù)* by Zhang Xi-Chun. Dr. Zhang posited that although the etiology and pathodynamic of irregular uterine bleeding is complicated, ultimately there is always damage to the Penetrating vessel and instability of qi transformation. Thus, one needs to urgently attend to the Penetrating vessel and to stabilize qi transformation. Dr. Zhang created two formulas: Quiet Gushing Decoction *(ān chōng tāng)* for light uterine bleeding and Stabilize Gushing Decoction *(gù chōng tāng)* for profuse uterine bleeding. However, after many attempts to use this approach, I found that Quiet Gushing Decoction *(ān chōng tāng)* worked acceptably for mild cases, but not for serious cases of light uterine bleeding. By serious cases, I mean that although the bleeding was light, it was very persistent and lasted for more than a month. For serious cases of light uterine bleeding, Stabilize Gushing Decoction *(gù chōng tāng)* produced better results. With regards to profuse uterine bleeding, I found that Stabilize Gushing Decoction *(gù chōng tāng)* was very quickly effective when it was given following the first episode of heavy bleeding. Its effects were much slower if there was a history of recurrent episodes of heavy bleeding.

Wistfully, I went back over the works of Dr. Zhang and unexpectedly found a postscript to Stabilize Gushing Decoction *(gù chōng tāng)* that sparked my interest:

> In *Fu Qing-Zhu Women's Disorders (Fù Qīng-Zhǔ nǚ kē)*, there is a formula for profuse uterine bleeding in elderly women that I tested and found to be very effective. The formula, called Modified Tangkuei Decoction to Tonify the Blood *(jiā jiǎn dāng guī bǔ xuè tāng)*, consists of Astragali Radix *(huáng qí)* (1 *liǎng*), wine-washed Angelicae sinensis Radix *(jiǔ xǐ dāng guī)* (1 *liǎng*), Mori Folium *(sāng yè)* (14 fresh leaves), powdered Notoginseng Radix *(sān qī)* (3 *qián* taken with the strained liquid). The formula is decocted in water. After two packets, the bleeding stops and after four packets it will not recur. If there is heat, it is suitable to add about 1 *liǎng* of Rehmanniae Radix *(shēng dì huáng)*.

The text continued, "This formula is also effective for young women."

At the time, I thought about this formula from Fu Qing-Zhu, which only has four ingredients and seems unremarkable; how could it be effective? However, I remembered that Zhang Xi-Chun was well-known for his innovation, his creativity, his emphasis on clinical practice, and his attention to clinical efficacy. He twice recommends the Fu Qing-Zhu text, which is unusual for him. If the efficacy of Modified Tangkuei Decoction to Tonify the Blood *(jiā jiǎn dāng guī bǔ xuè tāng)* was only about the same as Stabilize Gushing Decoction *(gù chōng tāng)*, why would he have bothered to recommend it twice?

Thus I made the decision to try the formula for some patients with severe irregular uterine bleeding. I found that it was very quickly effective for patients (within 2-4 packets the bleeding would stop) if they did not have qi stagnation and blood stasis. However, it was important to use the original formulation and the original dosages. For Mori Folium *(sāng yè)*, if the fresh leaves are unavailable, I use 30g of the dried leaves. Furthermore, regardless of whether or not there are heat signs, I add 30g of Rehmanniae Radix *(shēng dì huáng)* because it moderates the formula, which can then be used boldly and confidently. Finally, I was adamant about not adding any other medicinal substances to the formula.

PHYSICIAN B   Given that you have been using this formula for many years and that you have verified its efficacy, why have you not written an article about it before?

DR. YU   For many years I was unsure if it would be possible to replicate my results with this formula. When I began using this formula in the 70s, I was working in a mountain region. The women of these regions perform heavy labor and are susceptible to exhaustion of qi and blood. This formula greatly tonifies qi and blood, so of course it was effective for them. It was unclear to me if it would work as effectively for women in the lowlands and in urban areas.

Eventually, I was working in a prosperous lowland area and I met a mother and daughter who both reported profuse uterine bleeding. They had repeated episodes of profuse bleeding over a two-week period and Western medicine had not been effective. I gave them this formula and the bleeding stopped after two packets. In a short period of time, I then cured several other patients. My colleagues reacted with surprise, and also wanted to try this approach.

An example is Ms. Zhou, a 38-year-old woman with a constitutional tendency towards yin deficiency accompanied by dampness. She had a multi-year history of rheumatoid arthritis and had taken steroids over a long period of time. She had not had menstrual flow for three months (pregnancy had been ruled out) and then suddenly developed profuse bleeding which contained large clots. Because it was late in the day and she lived far away from my clinic, her husband hurriedly came to the clinic himself to ask for help. I sent him home with three packets of the formula and the bleeding stopped after the first packet. I have heard that since that time she has not had any recurrences.

Over the last few years, I have quickly cured many cases of urban women with severe irregular uterine bleeding using this formula. Now I am confident to recommend its use.

TREATMENT AND OUTCOME

■ CASE HISTORY 1

We prescribed the formula Modified Tangkuei Decoction to Tonify the Blood *(jiā jiǎn dāng guī bǔ xuè tāng)* with added Rehmanniae Radix *(shēng dì huáng)*:

Astragali Radix *(huáng qí)* 30g

wine-washed Angelicae sinensis Radix *(jiǔ xǐ dāng guī)* 30g

Mori Folium *(sāng yè)* 30g

Rehmanniae Radix *(shēng dì huáng)* 30g

powdered Notoginseng Radix *(sān qī)* 9g

    (taken with the cooked decoction 3g per dose, 3 times per day)

After one packet, the patient's bleeding decreased significantly, and after two packets, it stopped completely. Afterwards, we prescribed Black Chicken and White Phoenix Pill *(wū jī bái fèng wán)* and Restore the Spleen Decoction *(guī pí tāng)* for two months to regulate and tonify. For the next four years, her period was regular and she grew plump and robust. In mid-September 1989, following a period of overwork and fatigue, the patient's irregular uterine bleeding recurred. The blood volume increased day by day and after seven days it had not stopped. Two packets of the original formula were successful in stopping the bleeding. At that time, she had an ultrasound, which revealed the presence of a uterine fibroid. In November of the same year, she had a hysterectomy.

■ CASE HISTORY 2

Dr. Jiang had already prescribed a large packet of Tonify the Middle to Augment the Qi Decoction *(bǔ zhōng yì qì tāng)* combined with Flow-Warming Decoction *(wēn jīng tāng)*. In addition, he had instructed that 30g of Ginseng Radix *(rén shēn)* be made into a concentrated decoction that could be sipped frequently the moment that there was any more profuse bleeding. Coincidentally, I was present that day in the clinic and Dr. Jiang suggested that we first try the highly effective specialized formula that I knew for this situation. I prepared two formulas for the patient: #1. Modified Tangkuei Decoction to Tonify the Blood *(jiā jiǎn dāng guī bǔ xuè tāng)* with added Rehmanniae Radix *(shēng dì huáng)* in the same dosage and preparation as in the case above, and #2. Stabilize Gushing Decoction *(gù chōng tāng)*:

dry-fried Atractylodis macrocephalae Rhizoma *(chǎo bái zhú)* 30g

Astragali Radix *(huáng qí)* 18g

calcined Fossilia Ossis Mastodi *(duàn lóng gǔ)* 24g

calcined Ostreae Concha *(duàn mǔ lì)* 24g

Corni Fructus *(shān zhū yú)* 24g

Paeoniae Radix alba *(bái sháo)* 12g

Sepiae Endoconcha *(hǎi piāo xiāo)* 12g

Rubiae Radix *(qiàn cǎo gēn)* 9g

charred Trachycarpi Petiolus *(zōng lǘ tàn)* 6g

Galla chinensis *(wǔ bèi zǐ)* 1.5g

    (ground to a fine powder and taken with the cooked decoction—
    0.5g per dose, 3 times per day)

We instructed the patient to start with the first formula. If the bleeding decreased, she should then take all three packets to stop the bleeding. Afterward, if there was a small amount of bleeding, she could take four packets of Stabilize Gushing Decoction *(gù chōng tāng)* to deal with the remaining problem. If the first formula was ineffective, she should immediately change to the formula prepared by Dr. Jiang originally.

Ten days later, the patient's parents joyfully reported that after the first packet, the bleeding had abated significantly and that it had stopped completely by the time she finished the third packet. Two days later, there was a small amount of bleeding again, but one packet of Stabilize Gushing Decoction (gù chōng tāng) resolved that problem. She then finished all four packets of that formula. We recommended that she alternate Restore the Spleen Pill (guī pí wán) and Tonify the Middle to Augment the Qi Pill (bǔ zhōng yì qì wán) for one month to regulate and tonify.

At the time of this writing, Ms. You is a student at Leshan nursing school and for the two years following the treatment her periods have been completely normal. Furthermore, she gradually got healthier and stronger.

Disease	Primary symptoms	Differential diagnosis	Treatment method	Formula
Irregular uterine bleeding	Profuse, prolonged uterine bleeding	Exhaustion of qi and blood	Tonify the qi and contain the blood	Modified Tangkuei Decoction to Tonify the Blood (jiā jiǎn dāng guī bǔ xuè tāng)

REFLECTIONS AND CLARIFICATIONS

DR. YU   These two cases of irregular uterine bleeding were both serious, especially the second one. The patient was only 15 years old and because of the repeated profuse uterine bleeding and the failure of many different treatment approaches, the situation was becoming dire. Nonetheless, the bleeding was quickly controlled with Modified Tangkuei Decoction to Tonify the Blood (jiā jiǎn dāng guī bǔ xuè tāng) with added Rehmanniae Radix (shēng dì huáng).

After amassing many such cases, in recent years I have begun to consider this a specialized formula for the treatment of severe irregular uterine bleeding. My clinical experience has repeatedly confirmed that it is quickly effective for cases of severe irregular uterine bleeding, as long as the pattern does not involve qi stagnation or blood stasis.

PHYSICIAN A   According to textbooks, the etiology and pathology of irregular uterine bleeding can be divided into patterns such as blood heat, blood stasis, Spleen deficiency, and Kidney deficiency. Should we not differentiate patterns to determine treatment? Can one specialized formula be used for them all?

DR. YU   Although the causes and etiology of irregular uterine bleeding are varied, one can generalize by dividing the conditions into deficiency and excess. In clinic, once one clearly differentiates deficiency and excess, treatment can then be straightforward. In fact, clinical reasoning about this condition can be directly guided by thinking about specialized formulas for treatment. I would suggest that the Fu Qing-Zhu formula Modified Tangkuei Decoction to Tonify the Blood (jiā jiǎn dāng guī bǔ xuè tāng) treats severe patterns of deficiency-type irregular uterine bleeding.

PHYSICIAN B   What are the main indicators of severe patterns of deficiency-type irregular uterine bleeding?

<u>DR. YU</u>   In these patterns, the bleeding persists for a long time, the amount of blood lost is frightening, there may or may not be large blood clots, and abdominal pain is either very mild or nonexistent.

<u>PHYSICIAN C</u>   This is in regards to deficiency-type irregular uterine bleeding. There are other, more specific categories including qi deficiency, blood deficiency, and Kidney deficiency and the patient should be treated according to the presenting pattern.

<u>DR. YU</u>   This is the theoretical perspective, but clinically what we see is mixed patterns of deficiency with many symptoms, so it is difficult to draw sharp divisions or to force a patient into fitting one specific pattern. It is just as the common saying goes, "Memorizing the works of Wang Shu-He is not equal to rich clinical experience."[2]

My recommendation of this specialized formula does come with an additional consideration. In patterns of severe irregular uterine bleeding, because there is significant blood loss and great damage to the source qi, patients seeking help often have a great deal of anxiety about the situation. Thus, there is a need for the physician, after clearly establishing whether the pattern belongs to deficiency or excess, to utilize a highly effective formula. In this situation that means one that rapidly stops the bleeding without causing stasis and also nurtures and tonifies the source qi without resulting in stasis.

<u>PHYSICIAN A</u>   There is a journal that published a special discussion of "the differentiation and treatment of irregular uterine bleeding." The discussion represented a compilation of the experience of contemporary physicians in treating this condition. Other journals have also published work based on physician experience; so much has been published that it is hard to take it all in. And yet, in all that material, I have never seen a reference to the use of Modified Tangkuei Decoction to Tonify the Blood *(jiā jiǎn dāng guī bǔ xuè tāng)* with added Rehmanniae Radix *(shēng dì huáng)*. What is the mechanism behind the special efficacy of this formula?

<u>DR. YU</u>   The formula is composed of very commonplace ingredients that are nothing special. If you only take a general look at the formula and then proceed to a cursory explanation of its effects, it will be hard to convince people of its efficacy.

Fu Qing-Zhu explains that "Modified Tangkuei Decoction to Tonify the Blood *(jiā jiǎn dāng guī bǔ xuè tāng)* is a divine prescription for tonifying qi and blood. Notoginseng Radix *(sān qī)* is a sage-like herb for stopping bleeding. The addition of Mori Folium *(sāng yè)* enriches Kidney yin and also ingeniously restrains and inhibits."[3] Even if this explanation provides a plausible rationale for the formula's actions, it does not address a puzzling common question. Throughout the history of Chinese medicine, the formulas and herbs that tonify qi and blood, enrich Kidney yin, and restrain to stop

....

2. Wang Shu-He (180–270) was a physician who wrote the *Pulse Classic (mài jīng)*, an influential work describing pulse qualities and the importance of the pulse in diagnosis.

3. *Translators' note:* In earlier materia medica, such as the *Divine Husbandsman's Classic of the Materia Medica (Shén Nóng běn cǎo jīng)*, Mori Folium *(sāng yè)* is assigned functions that correlate with enriching yin, as well as restraining and inhibiting. Although these functions are often associated with the Liver, because the Liver and Kidney have the same source, these functions can also be thought of as influencing the Kidney yin.

bleeding are beyond counting. Are not all these other substances as effective as this formula?

Thus, I have always believed that whether discussing highly effective classical or contemporary formulas, the subtle details of the medicinal composition and dosage, as well as the chemical composition, must be considered essential information. It is still difficult to peer deeply into the subtle mysteries of these formulas.

Nonetheless, as a clinical physician, if one is able to start from the foundation of accurate pattern identification and knowledge of appropriate treatment methods, and then carefully sift through and test some highly effective specialized formulas, one day you will be able to confidently share this information with the medical world. This will allow others to easily use the formula effectively. Furthermore, it can be used to advance the process of research that should produce detailed and accurate clinical data. Is this not something worthwhile?

PHYSICIAN C   I noticed that in the first case, after the use of this formula, there was no recurrence of the bleeding for four years, but then the patient was diagnosed with a uterine fibroid and had no alternative but to have a hysterectomy. It appears that the formula is only useful for dysfunctional uterine bleeding.

DR. YU   I have used this formula to treat many cases of excessive bleeding resulting from uterine fibroids. Although the formula stops the bleeding quickly, recurrences happen easily. It seems likely that the presence of the fibroid, which is the root of the disease, is the main difficulty.

Nonetheless, our esteemed ancestors had a secret for a successful treatment strategy for uterine fibroids, which is "during the period, treat the excessive uterine bleeding, and after the period, treat the tumor." Although this formula cannot treat the tumor itself, it can temporarily stop the bleeding, which can alleviate some of the fear of more serious consequences and thus can be of some help in the process.

3.3 Breast lumps

Two cases of breast lumps

When seeking the root of a matter, investigate its true nature

追本溯源究 "实质"

■ CASE HISTORY 1

Patient No. 1: *30-year-old woman*

The patient presented with distending pain in both breasts that had persisted for two years. Palpation of the painful areas revealed a string of palpable small nodules that were pliable and tough, but not hard. The patient was diagnosed with lobular hyperplasia. She had taken a formula known as Reduce Breast Lumps *(rŭ kuài xiāo)*[4] (ten bottles, each of 500ml) that had reduced the distending pain significantly. However, not long afterward, following some upsetting events in her life, as her period approached, the distending pain returned. After that, she took more than 40 packets of a prescription combining Rambling Powder *(xiāo yáo săn)*, Two-Aged [Herb] Decoction *(èr chén tāng)*, and Bupleurum Powder to Dredge the Liver *(chái hú shū gān săn)*. While she was taking this prescription, her distending pain was reduced or eliminated, but as soon as her period approached, the pain returned.

INTAKE EXAMINATION
MARCH 21, 1986

The symptoms were as described above. Ordinarily, the patient experienced a feeling of fullness and a stifling sensation in her chest and diaphragm. She also reported epigastric and abdominal distention, belching, and a poor appetite. Her tongue was slightly pale and a little dusky with a thick, greasy, white coating. Her pulse was wiry and slippery.

■ CASE HISTORY 2

Patient No. 2: *42-year-old female*

This patient had an eight-month history of distending pain in both breasts. In the area around the breast an examining physician found extensive thin, flat, mobile nodules beneath the skin. She was diagnosed with lobular hyperplasia. She too had tried Reduce Breast Lumps *(rŭ kuài xiāo)* for two months. It had not brought any relief of her symptoms, but had caused her poor appetite, fatigue, and shortness of breath. She had also experimented on and off with modified versions of Augmented Rambling Powder *(jiā wèi xiāo yáo săn)* and Drive out Stasis from the Mansion of Blood Decoction *(xuè fŭ zhú yū tāng)*, but her symptoms remained the same.

INTAKE EXAMINATION
APRIL 10, 1987

The patient's complexion was pale, she was fatigued, her lumbosacral area was sore and painful, and she was irritable and easily angered. Her period was irregular, and her menstrual flow consisted of scanty, pale blood. The distending pain in her breasts was worse just prior to her menses. Her tongue was slightly pale with a thin, white coating and her pulse was wiry and weak.

DIFFERENTIATION OF PATTERNS AND DISCUSSION OF TREATMENT

PHYSICIAN A   The clinical manifestations of lobular hyperplasia are distending breast pain and the development of breast lumps. The Ming-dynasty physician Chen Shi-Gong is quoted in the *Orthodox Lineage of External Medicine (Wài kē zhèng zōng)* as saying:

....
4. Reduce Breast Lumps *(rŭ kuài xiāo)*: Citri reticulatae Folium *(jú yè)*, Salviae miltiorrhizae Radix *(dān shēn)*, Gleditsiae Spina *(zào jiăo cì)*, Vaccariae Semen *(wáng bù liú xíng)*, Toosendan Fructus *(chuān liàn zĭ)*, Pheretima *(dì lóng)*.

In cases of breast lumps and nodules within the breast that are egg-shaped, there may be a sinking heaviness that causes pain, or there may be no pain, and unaltered skin color. The nodules grow and shrink in conjunction with emotional changes. Many are the result of excessive thinking damaging the Spleen, and worry and frustration damaging the Liver. These [emotions] cause constraint and binding which produce [the lumps].

In Chinese medicine, this pattern is generally considered to be constrained and knotted Liver qi, possibly accompanied by phlegm congealing in the collaterals. Primary treatment relies on modifications of Rambling Powder *(xiāo yáo sǎn)* plus Two-Aged [Herb] Decoction *(èr chén tāng)* because of these formulas' ability to dredge the Liver qi, regulate qi, transform phlegm, and dispel stasis. If you can stick with this method and these formulas, especially in combination with psycho-emotional counseling, the treatment is relatively effective. In the two cases that are described above, the pathodynamic was like what I have described and yet the standard treatment was relatively ineffective. Does this simply reflect constitutional differences between individual patients?

DR. YU   Perhaps the difference actually lies in the pathodynamic. In the first case, the patient usually had fullness and a stifling sensation in her chest and diaphragm, distention in her epigastrium and abdomen, belching, poor appetite, a thick, white, greasy tongue coating, and a wiry and slippery pulse. These symptoms are characteristic of Liver constraint, clogged Stomach, congealed phlegm, and qi stagnation, which is quite different from simply constrained and knotted Liver qi. This difference is even more pronounced in the second case, in which the patient was perimenopausal and had Kidney deficiency and Liver constraint.

   The first case was treated with a modification of Zhang Jing-Yue's Resolve the Liver Decoction *(jiě gān jiān).*[5] This formula relieves Liver constraint, resolves a clogged Stomach, transforms phlegm, and directs rebellious qi downward. After the local and systemic symptoms had improved, we added medicinal substances to invigorate the blood, unblock the collaterals, soften hardness, and disperse knots, along with a large dosage of Astragali Radix *(huáng qí)* to support the normal qi. In this way, we were able to reduce and dissipate phlegm and blood stasis without damaging the normal qi.

TREATMENT AND OUTCOME

■ CASE HISTORY 1

After careful thought we considered this to be a pattern of Liver constraint and clogged Stomach with phlegm congealing in the Stomach collaterals. The treatment principle was to dredge Liver qi, harmonize the Stomach, transform phlegm, and unblock the collaterals. We chose a modification of Resolve the Liver Decoction *(jiě gān jiān)* from Zhang Jing-Yue:

standard Pinelliae Rhizoma praeparatum *(fǎ bàn xià)* 15g
Magnoliae officinalis Cortex *(hòu pò)* 20g

....

5. Resolve the Liver Decoction *(jiě gān jiān)* is a combination of Pinellia and Magnolia Bark Decoction *(bàn xià hòu pò tāng)* and Two-Aged [Herb] Decoction *(èr chén tāng)* plus Amomi Fructus *(shā rén)* and Paeoniae Radix alba *(bái sháo).*

Perillae Caulis *(zǐ sū gěng)* 15g

Poria *(fú líng)* 20g

Zingiberis Rhizoma recens *(shēng jiāng)* 10g

Amomi Fructus *(shā rén)* 6g

Citri reticulatae Pericarpium *(chén pí)* 15g

Sargassum *(hǎi zǎo)* 30g

Eckloniae Thallus *(kūn bù)* 30g

untreated Glycyrrhizae Radix *(shēng gān cǎo)* 12g

Instructions: Six packets were prescribed.

SECOND VISIT: The patient reported a marked reduction in breast distention and pain, stifling sensation in the chest, and abdominal distention. However, during her period, her breast distention and pain increased. Her menstrual blood was dark brown and contained clots.

To the above formula, I added:

pearls of Manitis Squama *(chuān shān jiǎ zhū)* 10g

Lycopi Herba *(zé lán)* 15g

Cyathulae Radix *(chuān niú xī)* 15g

Astragali Radix *(huáng qí)* 30g

Sparganii Rhizoma *(sān léng)* 15g

Curcumae Rhizoma *(é zhú)* 15g

Instructions: Six packets were prescribed.

She was also prescribed Flecks of Gold Tabs *(xiǎo jīn piàn)*[6] at a dosage of four pills, three times per day for the following two months.

After taking six packets of the formula, the patient's breast distention and pain had resolved. I directed her to take three more packets during the next premenstrual phase of her cycle. When her period arrived, it flowed easily, the color was normal, and there were no clots. However, she needed to continue on Minor Metal Pill *(xiǎo jīn piàn)* for a full three months before her breast nodules disappeared completely. Follow-up for the next two years revealed no recurrences.

■ CASE HISTORY 2

We considered this to be a pattern of Kidney deficiency and Liver constraint with phlegm congealing in the Stomach collaterals. It is appropriate to start with attending to the root by tonifying the Kidney and dredging the Liver. I chose a modification of the combination of Two-Immortal Decoction *(èr xiān tāng)* and Settle the Menses Decoction *(dìng jīng tāng)*.[7]

....

6. *Translators' note:* Flecks of Gold Tabs (小金片 *xiǎo jīn piàn*) is a modern patent formula based on a formula of the same name from the Qing-dynasty text *Complete Compendium of Patterns and Treatments in External Medicine (Wài kē zhèng zhì quán shēng jí)*. It includes Momordicae Semen *(mù biē zǐ)*, Aconiti kusnezoffii Radix praeparata *(zhì cǎo wū)*, Liquidambaris Resina *(fēng xiāng zhī)*, Olibanum *(rǔ xiāng)*, Myrrha *(mò yào)*, Trogopterori Faeces *(wǔ líng zhī)*, Angelicae sinensis Radix *(dāng guī)*, Pheretima *(dì lóng)*, and ink from an ink stick. At present it is used for a few types of cancer, yin toxic swellings, nodules, etc.

7. Settle the Menses Decoction (定經湯 *dìng jīng tāng*) from *Fu Qing-Zhu's Women's Disorders*

Curculiginis Rhizoma *(xiān máo)* 15g

Epimedii Herba *(yín yáng huò)* 30g

Morindae officinalis Radix *(bā jǐ tiān)* 15g

Cervi Cornu degelatinatum *(lù jiǎo shuāng)* 15g

Rehmanniae Radix praeparata *(shú dì huáng)* 30g

Cuscutae Semen *(tù sī zǐ)* 15g

Bupleuri Radix *(chái hú)* 10g

Schizonepetae Herba *(jīng jiè)* 6g

Dioscoreae Rhizoma *(shān yào)* 15g

Poria *(fú líng)* 30g

Angelicae sinensis Radix *(dāng guī)* 12g

Paeoniae Radix alba *(bái sháo)* 12g

Instructions: ten packets were prescribed.

SECOND VISIT: The patient's spirit and complexion had improved significantly. Her lumbo-sacral pain had declined and she was less irritable and less easily angered. The distending pain in her breasts had also decreased. To the previous formula, we added medicinal substances to transform phlegm, soften hardness, and unblock the collaterals:

Curculiginis Rhizoma *(xiān máo)* 15g

Epimedii Herba *(yín yáng huò)* 30g

Morindae officinalis Radix *(bā jǐ tiān)* 15g

Cervi Cornu degelatinatum *(lù jiǎo shuāng)* 15g

Bupleuri Radix *(chái hú)* 10g

Paeoniae Radix alba *(bái sháo)* 12g

Angelicae sinensis Radix *(dāng guī)* 12g

Scrophulariae Radix *(xuán shēn)* 15g

Fritillariae thunbergii Bulbus *(zhè bèi mǔ)* 20g

Ostreae Concha *(mǔ lì)* 30g

pearls of Manitis squama *(chuān shān jiǎ zhū)* 10g

Bombyx batryticatus *(bái jiāng cán)* 10g

Vespae Nidus *(lù fēng fáng)* 10g

Instructions: Fifteen packets were prescribed.

After finishing 15 packets, the patient's distending breast pain and breast lumps had resolved. Her menses was essentially normal. One-year follow-up revealed no recurrence.

REFLECTIONS AND CLARIFICATIONS

PHYSICIAN E Dr. Yu, in both of these cases we include pearls of Manitis Squama *(chuān shān jiǎ zhū)*. This item derives from an endangered species and is no longer in use. Do you have a suggestion for substituting for this medicinal substance?

DR. YU Yes, in recent years this item is not available for use. Certainly, pearls of Manitis

---

(Fù Qīng-Zhǔ nǚ kē): wine-fried Cuscutae Semen *(jiǔ chǎo tù sī zǐ)*, wine-fried Paeoniae Radix alba *(jiǔ chǎo bái sháo)*, wine-washed Angelicae sinensis Radix *(jiǔ xǐ dāng guī)*, Rehmanniae Radix praeparata *(shú dì huáng)*, Dioscoreae Rhizoma *(shān yào)*, Poria *(fú líng)*, Blackened Schizonepetae Spica *(chǎo hēi jīng jiè suì)*, Bupleuri Radix *(chái hú)*.

Squama *(chuān shān jiǎ zhū)* have a special property. They can penetrate, attack hardness, unblock the collaterals, and break up accumulations. They have the power to do this while at the same time not injuring normal qi. There are no plant-based substances that have this unique nature. Nonetheless, nowadays I rely on the three-herb combination of Angelicae dahuricae Radix *(bái zhǐ)* 15g, Gleditsiae Spina *(zào jiǎo cì)* 10g, and Vaccariae Semen *(wáng bù liú xíng)* 30g as a substitute for pearls of Manitis Squama *(chuān shān jiǎ zhū)*.

PHYSICIAN B   The second patient was a middle-aged woman with irregular periods and increasingly severe distending breast pain. Additionally, she had lumbosacral soreness and pain. She was irritable and easily angered. This pattern is obviously an imbalance between the Penetrating and Conception vessels. Previous physicians had mostly prescribed formulas to dredge the Liver and regulate the qi, and to invigorate the blood and transform stasis, with poor results. I observed that upon receiving this patient for treatment you decided to make a fresh start and changed to a modified combination of Two-Immortal Decoction *(èr xiān tāng)* and Settle the Menses Decoction *(dìng jīng tāng)*. Obviously, this approach is primarily regulating the Penetrating and Conception vessels. The treatment went unchanged for an extended time because the improvement was gradual. However, in the discussion of the diagnosis, you mentioned Kidney deficiency and Liver constraint, completely avoiding any mention of an imbalance between the Penetrating and Conception vessels. What is your rationale?

DR. YU   If you attribute these symptoms to the abstract diagnosis of an 'imbalance between the Penetrating and Conception vessels,' then there will be no true way to find a treatment.

PHYSICIAN B   Why is that?

DR. YU   The Penetrating and Conception vessels are among the eight extraordinary vessels. In Chapter 1 of *Basic Questions (Sū wèn)* it states that, "When the Conception vessel is unblocked and the Great Penetrating vessel is filled, the menses arrives." Later generations have added that the "Penetrating vessel is the sea of blood" and "the Conception vessel governs the Womb and the fetus." Therefore, to attribute menstrual irregularity to an imbalance between the Penetrating and Conception vessels is not without a certain logic. The practical problem is that this pathodynamic does not lead to a specific formula or group of medicinal substances.

Chapter 33 of the *Divine Pivot (Líng shū)* states, "The 12 channels interiorly pertain to the organs and exteriorly connect to the limbs and joints." The foundation of the functional activity of the channels and collaterals resides in the yin and yang organs. If separated from the organs, the channels no longer have an existence. Furthermore, the Penetrating and Conception vessels belong to the eight extraordinary channels; they are not part of the system of the 12 regular channels and so there is no way for them to communicate directly with the organs. To put it another way, only by passing through the 12 regular channels can the fine essence of the organs then indirectly reach the Penetrating and Conception vessels. The same is true for pathological changes. Therefore, an imbalance between the Penetrating and Conception vessels is a disease manifestation in which an imbalance of the organs is the root.

In addition, from a clinical perspective, can I ask what group of medicinal substances directly treats an imbalance between the Penetrating and Conception vessels? I'm afraid that this question is very difficult to answer. One of the reasons for this difficulty is that when we talk about the entering channels of medicinal substances, none is said to go to the Penetrating and Conception vessels.

The famous early 20th-century physician Zhang Xi-Chun relied heavily on the Penetrating vessel when treating menstrual irregularity. He created the well-known formulas Regulate Gushing Decoction *(lǐ chōng tāng)*, Calm Gushing Decoction *(ān chōng tāng)*, and Stabilize Gushing Decoction *(gù chōng tāng)*.[8] However, if we consider carefully the medicinal substances in his formulas, such as Astragali Radix *(huáng qí)*, Atractylodis macrocephalae Rhizoma *(bái zhú)*, Paeoniae Radix alba *(bái sháo)*, Corni Fructus *(shān zhū yú)*, Dipsaci Radix *(xù duàn)*, Fossilia Ossis Mastodi *(lóng gǔ)*, Ostreae Concha *(mǔ lì)*, Sepiae Endoconcha *(hǎi piāo xiāo)*, Rubiae Radix *(qiàn cǎo gēn)*, Sparganii Rhizoma *(sān léng)*, Curcumae Rhizoma *(é zhú)*, Gigeriae galli Endothelium corneum *(jī nèi jīn)*, and Hirudo *(shuǐ zhì)*, we find that they all belong to categories of herbs such as substances that strengthen the Spleen and augment the qi, secure the Kidney qi, and invigorate the blood and transform stasis. Thus, in fact, they are all regulating the Spleen, Liver, and Kidney. It is only because of this that the treatments have an effect.

In perusing modern and ancient treatments for lobular hyperplasia, those who take delight in extolling "regulating the Penetrating and Conception vessels" are really quite rare! Thus, when we hear popular platitudes in medicine, it is important to integrate them with the realities of clinical practice so that we acquire a firm grasp of their true meaning.

PHYSICIAN B   Is lobular hyperplasia from Kidney deficiency and Liver constraint a commonly seen pattern in the clinic?

DR. YU   That pattern is unquestionably more common in perimenopausal women. However overall, it is still true that the most common pattern for this disorder is constrained and knotted Liver qi. My reason for bringing up two less frequently seen patterns in those with lobular hyperplasia (Liver constraint and clogged Stomach along with Kidney deficiency and Liver constraint) is to help practitioners avoid a common tendency that can occur in those with copious clinical experience: upon seeing lobular hyperplasia, they immediately attribute it to constrained and knotted Liver qi, and without proper thought, prescribe a prepared medicine.

PHYSICIAN B   Both of the patients you described had taken Reduce Breast Lumps *(rǔ kuài xiāo)* and its effects were either nonexistent or short-lived. This outcome suggests the importance of differentiating patterns to determine treatment and reminds me that we should not automatically rely on pre-made formulations of medicinal substances. However, given that this medicinal substance mixture has a high rate of efficacy in treating lobular hyperplasia, I am interested to know about the specific medicinal substances in the formula.

....

8. *Translators' note:* The word 衝 *chōng*, which we have translated as 'gushing' in the names of these formulas, can also refer to the 衝脈 *chōng mài*—the Penetrating vessel.

DR. YU   As far as I know, the 'orthodox' formulation of Reduce Breast Lumps Mixture *(rǔ kuài xiāo)* was created in the Dongzhimen affiliated hospital of the Beijing College of Traditional Chinese Medicine. The formula consists of Salviae miltiorrhizae Radix *(dān shēn)* 15g, Citri reticulatae Semen *(jú hé)* 15g, Vaccariae Semen *(wáng bù liú xíng)* 10g, Toosendan Fructus *(chuān liàn zǐ)* 10g, Eupolyphaga/Stelophaga *(tǔ biē chóng)* 10g, and Gleditsiae Spina *(zào jiǎo cì)* 10g. In my experience, if the administration of a few packets of this formula is ineffective, one can change to Reduce Nodules Decoction *(xiāo hé tāng)*, which was introduced by the famous modern physician Zhu Liang-Chun and is composed of prepared Bombyx batryticatus *(zhì bái jiāng cán)* 12g, Vespae Nidus *(lù fēng fáng)* 9g, Angelicae sinensis Radix *(dāng guī)* 9g, Paeoniae Radix rubra *(chì sháo)* 9g, Cyperi Rhizoma *(xiāng fù)* 9g, Citri reticulatae Semen *(jú hé)* 9g, Citri reticulatae Pericarpium *(chén pí)* 6g, Glycyrrhizae Radix *(gān cǎo)* 3g. If the patient is also willing to engage in psychological counseling, a positive outcome is more likely.

PHYSICIAN A   In the standard list of the 18 incompatibilities, Sargassum *(hǎi zǎo)* is incompatible with Glycyrrhizae Radix *(gān cǎo)*. In the formula for the first patient, these two medicinal substances are used together. Isn't this pairing considered problematic?

DR. YU   In reviewing classical literature, early on we encounter the 18 incompatibilities (十八反 *shí bā fǎn*) of materia medica that should not be combined.[9] For example, Kansui Radix *(gān suì)* is incompatible with Glycyrrhizae Radix *(gān cǎo)*. However, Kansui and Pinellia Decoction *(gān suì bàn xià tāng)*, from the *Essentials of the Golden Cabinet (Jīn guì yào lüè)*, which is used to treat lodged thin mucus, contains this combination. The famous Jin-dynasty physician Li Dong-Yuan also makes uses of this combination in some of his formulas. Another example is the incompatibility between Aconiti Radix praeparata *(zhì* chuān *wū)* and Pinelliae Rhizoma praeparatum *(zhì bàn xià)*. The Red Pill *(chì wán)*[10] from *Essentials of the Golden Cabinet (Jīn guì yào lüè)*, which treats cold qi reversal counterflow, makes use of this combination.

We can see that ancient physicians were not handcuffed by the 18 incompatibilities, even though they were discussed in the materia medica of the time. Practitioners of later generations were even less restrained. It has become common practice for contemporary physicians to report on the effective use of Kansui Radix *(gān suì)* and Glycyrrhizae Radix *(gān cǎo)*, Aconiti Radix praeparata *(zhì* chuān *wū)* and Pinelliae Rhizoma praeparatum *(zhì bàn xià)*, and Sargassum *(hǎi zǎo)* and Glycyrrhizae Radix *(gān cǎo)*.

With regards to the 19 antagonisms (十九畏 *shí jiǔ wèi*) of the materia medica, these represent another set of medicinal substance incompatibilities. An example is the antagonism between Caryophylli Flos *(dīng xiāng)* and Curcumae Radix *(yù jīn)*. Yet modern physicians readily use this combination for its quick effect in eliminating

....

9. *Translators' note:* This list of substances that are considered incompatible goes back to the early 13th-century work, *Confucians' Duties to Their Parents (Rú mén shì qīn)* by Zhang Cong-Zheng.

10. The Red Pill *(chì wán)* includes Poria *(fú líng)*, Pinelliae Rhizoma praeparatum *(zhì bàn xià)*, Aconiti Radix praeparata *(zhì* chuān *wū)*, and Asari Radix et Rhizoma *(xì xīn)*. This combination of herbs is ground to a powder, a bit of Cinnabar *(zhū shā)* is added, and the powder is mixed with honey to make small pills the size of hemp seeds. The red color added to the formula by the inclusion of cinnabar makes the pill red, thus the appellation.

qi stagnation in the chest and diaphragm. Another example is the antagonism between Ginseng Radix *(rén shēn)* and Trogopterori Faeces *(wǔ líng zhī)*. This combination is, however, frequently used for its ability to tonify qi and transform stasis in patterns that combine qi deficiency and blood stasis.

It is important to remember that modern physicians not only do extensive clinical testing of medicinal substances and formulas, but also make use of modern pharmacologic methods for verifying the results. The 18 incompatibilities and 19 antagonisms of the traditional materia medica have no scientific basis. As the ancient poem says, "Please do not play the tunes of former dynasties, let's listen to the singing of a new melody made for today." We are modern physicians and we should have the courage to face modern reality. We should cultivate the ability to assimilate new concepts and new understandings arising from testing and examination.

To return to the main topic, Sargassum *(hǎi zǎo)* is very useful in the treatment of lobular hyperplasia. The entry from the *Divine Husbandsman's Classic of the Materia Medica (Shén Nóng běn cǎo jīng)* states that it "governs goiters, tumors, and knotted qi, as well as nodules in the lower area of the neck. It breaks up knots and disperses qi, treats abscesses and swellings, abdominal masses, and firm qi." If we can draw lessons from the thought process of contemporary physicians, it seems that the pairing of Sargassum *(hǎi zǎo)* and Glycyrrhizae Radix *(gān cǎo)* is quickly effective and without side effects.

Perhaps this pairing should be considered opposing yet complementary. To further elaborate, in recent years I have treated many patients with thyroid tumors and uterine fibroids in which the main diagnosis or an important component of the diagnosis was congealing of stubborn phlegm. To appropriate formulas used for these conditions, I have often added Sargassum *(hǎi zǎo)* and Glycyrrhizae Radix *(gān cǎo)* and it has never let me down.

3.4 Postpartum diseases

Three cases: postpartum insufficiency of breast milk, postpartum overflow of breast milk, postpartum constipation

Deeply investigate the pathodynamic: different diseases can be treated similarly.

深研病机：異病同治

■ CASE HISTORY 1

Insufficient lactation in a 28-year-old female

The patient had experienced a full-term pregnancy with a smooth vaginal delivery two months previous. Her breast milk was insufficient and her appetite was poor. After giving birth, she ate the traditional post-childbirth diet of pig trotters, peanuts, and cuttlefish stew for a few days, but it did not help and her appetite diminished further. She was given three packets of a formula containing Manitis Squama *(chuān shān jiǎ)*, Vaccariae Semen *(wáng bù liú xíng)*, Angelicae sinensis Radix *(dāng guī)*, and Astragali Radix *(huáng qí)* but the volume of her milk was still insufficient. Further treatment with a formula containing Cyperi Rhizoma *(xiāng fù)*, Linderae Radix *(wū yào)*, Toosendan Fructus *(chuān liàn zǐ)*, Bupleuri Radix *(chái hú)*, Curcumae Radix *(yù jīn)*, and Magnoliae officinalis Cortex *(hòu pò)* was also ineffective.

INTAKE EXAMINATION
OCTOBER 25, 1985

Both of the patient's breasts were slightly distended. Her appetite was poor and she complained of belching and a stifling sensation in her chest. Her tongue was a pale red with a thin, yellow coating. Her pulse was wiry, fine, and slightly tight. Upon further questioning, she revealed that after delivery, she had experienced some disagreeable situations and been unable to express her feelings about them.

■ CASE HISTORY 2

25-year-old female with postpartum overflow of breast milk

The patient's full-term pregnancy ended with a smooth vaginal delivery. When she began breastfeeding, her newborn spit out the first and second mouthfuls of breast milk. After that, her infant refused to feed and would begin crying if forced. The patient was curious about this and so tasted her breast milk. She found it to have a peculiar taste, which was confirmed by a friend, who also tasted it. She decided to stop breastfeeding and wanted to get the flow of breast milk to stop. At first, she used 120g of dry-fried Hordei Fructus germinatus *(chǎo mài yá)* decocted once a day for three days, but this had no effect on her breast milk, nor did several packets of a folk remedy for reducing breast milk flow, which she took several times.

A physician suggested that following delivery, qi and blood were deficient and so prescribed Tangkuei Decoction to Tonify the Blood *(dāng guī bǔ xuè tāng)* and then All-Inclusive Great Tonifying Decoction *(shí quán dà bǔ tāng)*, three packets each, but the overflowing breast milk remained unchanged. Another physician suggested that her Kidneys were deficient and so prescribed Kidney tonics, while still another suggested that she suffered from heat in the blood and prescribed a formula to cool the blood. Over the course of six months she took between 50-60 packets of Chinese herbal formulas, but her symptoms remained unchanged.

INTAKE EXAMINATION
OCTOBER 25, 1985

Milk was constantly dripping out of her breasts. She covered her breasts with a thick towel and in about an hour, the milk would saturate the towel. This meant that she had to repeatedly replace the towel during the day. Other than this, her complexion and appetite were good, and her pulse and tongue showed no signs of illness.

■ CASE HISTORY 3

26-year-old female with postpartum constipation

The patient had a full-term pregnancy with a Caesarean delivery. Since the delivery she has been continually constipated. At first, Hemp Seed Pill *(má zǐ rén wán)* was effective in relieving the symptoms, but after ten days of administration, its efficacy diminished. She then tried phenolphthalein tablets and an enema. When she did not have a bowel movement for five or six days and experienced unbearable abdominal distention, she would take Sennae Folium *(fān xiè yè)* as a purgative. This problem had been going on for more than three months.

INTAKE EXAMINATION
OCTOBER 26, 1985

She reported abdominal distention and flatulence. Her tongue was pale red with a thin, white coating that lacked moisture. Her pulse was wiry and fine.

DIFFERENTIATION OF PATTERNS AND DISCUSSION OF TREATMENT

PHYSICIAN A   In Chapter 39 of the *Basic Questions (Sū wèn)* it states, "The hundred diseases arise in relation to qi." Physicians over the years have explained this by saying that if qi and blood are flowing and harmonious, no disease will arise. However, as soon as there is constraint, the hundred diseases will arise.

When qi and blood move counter to normal flow or become constrained, the responsibility lies with a loss of the Liver's ability to drain and disperse and to thrust outward. When this occurs, the Liver will exploit the Spleen and accost the Stomach. In this way, a pathodynamic of qi stagnation affecting the Liver and Stomach can appear or be concealed within many different disease states. This situation does not seem difficult to explain. Would you agree?

DR. YU   This basic idea is in accordance with the principles of medicine, but your wording is imprecise. The pathodynamic represents the inherent mechanism of a disease process, how can it be said "to appear?" What appears are the symptoms of the disease, whereas the pathodynamic always resides within the disease itself. It is necessary for physicians to utilize abstract thinking to analyze, induce, deduce, and synthesize.

The *Inner Classic (Nèi jīng)* admonishes physicians to deeply investigate the pathodynamic; Chapter 74 of *Basic Questions (Sù wèn)* states, "When [signs and symptoms] are present, investigate them. When [signs and symptoms] are absent, investigate them." The meaning is that we must seek to understand the pathodynamic whether or not there are clearly related clinical symptoms.

In Case 1, where there is insufficient breast milk, the patient had experienced some unresolved difficult life situations. We can deduce that there was a pattern of Liver-Stomach qi stagnation.

In Case 2, where there is overflowing breast milk, does the patient have a disease? Although there do not appear to be any systemic problems, there is a local symptom, which is that the mother's breast milk will not stop flowing. The breast belongs to the

Stomach channel and the nipple belongs to the Liver channel. The fact that the breast milk had a strange taste and that the flow would not cease indicates that there is a failure of the normal processes in the area where the qi and blood of the Liver and Stomach are concentrated. This failure has continued for over six months, and the use of formulas that tonify qi and blood, those that tonify the Liver and Kidneys, as well as those that clear heat and cool the blood were all ineffective. Given this state of affairs, it is natural that one would shift to considering the pathodynamic to be an obstruction of the qi dynamic associated with the Liver and Stomach. This is often present yet frequently overlooked.

TREATMENT AND OUTCOME

■ CASE HISTORY 1

This case belongs to a pattern in which the Liver is constrained and not soothed. The standard formulas for unblocking the flow of breast milk were ineffective. After giving her some advice about her emotional state, I prescribed a modification of Frigid Extremities Powder *(sì nì sǎn)*:

Bupleuri Radix *(chái hú)*	10g
Paeoniae Radix alba *(bái sháo)*	15g
dry-fried Aurantii Fructus *(chǎo zhǐ ké)*	10g
untreated Glycyrrhizae Radix *(shēng gān cǎo)*	6g
Moutan Cortex *(mǔ dān pí)*	6g
vinegar-processed Cyperi Rhizoma *(cù zhì xiāng fù)*	10g

After three packets, the patient's breast distention had disappeared and the volume of her breast milk had increased. To this formula, I added Astragali Radix *(huáng qí)* 15g and Angelicae sinensis Radix *(dāng guī)* 6g. She continued taking six more packets and her breast milk gradually increased to the point that it was sufficient for nursing her baby.

■ CASE HISTORY 2

How is one to differentiate the pattern in this case? After much deliberation, I decided to prescribe Frigid Extremities Powder *(sì nì sǎn)* with a large dosage of Corni Fructus *(shān zhū yú)*.

Bupleuri Radix *(chái hú)*	10g
Paeoniae Radix alba *(bái sháo)*	15g
dry-fried Aurantii Fructus *(chǎo zhǐ ké)*	10g
untreated Glycyrrhizae Radix *(shēng gān cǎo)*	5g
Corni Fructus *(shān zhū yú)*	30g

I advised her to try two packets and then return to the clinic. After three days, she returned with a big smile on her face saying that after finishing two packets, the flow of breast milk had been reduced by more than half. She continued this formula, but with the addition of Astragali Radix *(huáng qí)* 30g, calcined Fossilia Ossis Mastodi *(duàn lóng gǔ)* 30g, and calcined Ostreae Concha *(duàn mǔ lì)* 30g.

After three more packets, unexpectedly, the flow of breast milk returned to its previous volume. I advised her to go back to using the original formula. If it did not work, she was told to return to the clinic so that we could change the formula.

Two months later she returned to the clinic for treatment of a different complaint. She reported that after taking eight packets of the formula, the flow of breast milk ceased completely and her breasts returned to normal.

■ CASE HISTORY 3

Because it was autumn, I thought that Lung-metal was harshly overwhelming Liver-wood. It was appropriate to clarify the Lung, soothe the Liver, and gently moisten the Intestines in order to unblock the stool. I prescribed an augmented version of Frigid Extremities Powder *(sì nì sǎn)*:

Bupleuri Radix *(chái hú)*	10g
Paeoniae Radix alba *(bái sháo)*	30g
dry-fried Aurantii Fructus *(chǎo zhǐ ké)*	15g
Glycyrrhizae Radix *(gān cǎo)*	6g
Armeniacae Semen *(xìng rén)*	15g
Eriobotryae Folium *(pí pá yè)*	30g
prepared Asteris Radix *(zhì zǐ wǎn)*	30g

After taking one packet, the patient's bowels were unblocked and her abdominal distention and flatulence significantly decreased. She continued taking this formula, one packet every two days, for 12 days. Her stool was then normal and no recurrence was reported on a follow-up two months later.

REFLECTIONS AND CLARIFICATIONS

PHYSICIAN B   Although the symptoms of postpartum breast milk insufficiency and breast milk overflow are exactly the opposite, in this case the pathodynamic for both is the same: qi stagnation affecting the Liver and Stomach. Chinese medicine treatment is directed at the pathodynamic; thus, we can apply different treatments to the same disease and different diseases may be treated with the same treatment.

One thing that seems worth contemplating is that in the case of insufficient breast milk, the patient had tried medicinal substances to dredge the Liver and move the qi. Why do you think those medicinal substances were ineffective, while Frigid Extremities Powder *(sì nì sǎn)*, which has the same actions, was so effective?

DR. YU   The pattern differentiation for postpartum breast milk insufficiency was Liver-Stomach qi stagnation; therefore, the correct treatment was to dredge the Liver and move the qi. But I must confess that when thinking about which Liver-dredging and qi-moving formula to use, there are many that can be considered. Ultimately, which formula will be most effective? This decision will differ from patient to patient.

In this case of breast milk insufficiency resulting from Liver and Stomach qi stagnation, Frigid Extremities Powder *(sì nì sǎn)* was highly effective and the other formulas were not; this reflects individual differences among patients. Consideration of the individual differences among patients is one of the distinguishing features of Chinese medicine. This aspect of Chinese medicine has already spread into the world of Western medicine. For example, experienced Western medicine physicians, when prescribing antibiotics, will choose not only a primary drug, but a secondary and tertiary choice. They will not hang all their hopes on one. Is this not also paying attention to individual differences?

In recent years, when addressing difficult diseases, I have advocated that Chinese medicine practitioners, once they have established an accurate pattern differentiation and treatment principle, seek out highly effective formulas. If you have not mastered what a highly effective formula would be in a certain situation, then you should advance step by step through primary, secondary, and tertiary formulas, striving for optimal efficacy. In this way, you can avoid the trap of being a practitioner with a single insight who then becomes stuck in indecision should a tried and true formula fail to work. You can end up having no clear understanding of the situation and nowhere to turn. Where the medicine and the disease pattern don't match, it is not difficult to end up with an intractable disease.

PHYSICIAN B   In the second case, in which the patient's breast milk was overflowing, the woman was healthy and there were no obvious signs of qi stagnation affecting the Liver and Stomach. How is it that you chose Frigid Extremities Powder *(sì nì sǎn)* with a large dosage of Corni Fructus *(shān zhū yú)* for her and achieved such quick results? Also, why did the overflowing breast milk return after you added Astragali Radix *(huáng qí)*, calcined Fossilia Ossis Mastodi *(duàn lóng gǔ)*, and calcined Ostreae Concha *(duàn mǔ lì)* to the formula?

DR. YU   To this day, I cannot claim to fully understand the subtleties of this case, so all I can do is to present a relatively superficial explanation. With regards to overflowing breast milk in postpartum women, I remembered that qi stagnation affecting the Liver and Stomach is a commonly occurring, but frequently overlooked, disease dynamic. Thus, I thought to try Frigid Extremities Powder *(sì nì sǎn)*, which dredges the Liver and harmonizes the Stomach. I employed a large dosage of Corni Fructus *(shān zhū yú)*, which, being sour, preserves Liver yin and offers a balance to the base formula which unblocks and spreads out the Liver qi by being sour. This combination creates a balance between opening and closing. I honestly was not certain if this would be sufficient to stop the outflow of milk.

After taking the formula, the overflowing breast milk was reduced by more than half and I should have simply continued with this course of action. However, I remembered the admonition of Zhu Dan-Xi regarding postpartum patients: the first course of action should be to strongly tonify the qi and blood, even if other symptoms are present. This recollection led me to make the mistake of adding Astragali Radix *(huáng qí)*, calcined Fossilia Ossis Mastodi *(duàn lóng gǔ)*, and calcined Ostreae Concha *(duàn mǔ lì)*, thereby temporarily damaging the efficacy of the formula.

PHYSICIAN B   The first two cases, treated on the same day, presented with precisely opposite complaints: one with insufficiency of breast milk and the other with overflowing breast milk, yet they were both treated effectively with the same formula, Frigid Extremities Powder *(sì nì sǎn)*.

This is unfathomable. Frigid Extremities Powder *(sì nì sǎn)* is composed of Bupleuri Radix *(chái hú)*, Paeoniae Radix alba *(bái sháo)*, Aurantii Fructus immaturus *(zhǐ shí)* (or Aurantii Fructus *[zhǐ ké]*) and Glycyrrhizae Radix *(gān cǎo)*. It is intriguing that you were able to use this formula with its four very ordinary medicinal substances, through skillful modification, to such extraordinary effect. We have since browsed through your unpublished cases and discovered many cases that were treated effectively with this formula. Furthermore, its range of application is quite broad, touching on all branches of practice including gynecology, pediatrics, internal medicine, external medicine, ophthalmology and ear, nose, and throat disorders. Now, having presented us with three postpartum cases in which Frigid Extremities Powder *(sì nì sǎn)* was surprisingly effective, we are interested to discuss this topic more deeply.

DR. YU   Frigid Extremities Powder *(sì nì sǎn)* is a common formula for dredging the Liver and harmonizing the Stomach. The fact that this classical formula is applicable to such a wide range of cases in modern clinical practice illustrates that the underlying pathodynamic, qi constraint affecting the Liver and Stomach, is a component of many different disorders. The *Golden Mirror of the Medical Tradition (Yī zōng jīn jiàn)* explains the formula as follows:

> The chief herb, Bupleuri Radix *(chái hú)*, dredges Liver yang, the deputy herb, Paeoniae Radix *(sháo yào)*, drains Liver yin, the assistant herb, Glycyrrhizae Radix *(gān cǎo)*, moderates Liver qi, and the envoy herb, Aurantii Fructus immaturus *(zhǐ shí)*, directs counterflow qi downward. In the presence of Bupleuri Radix *(chái hú)*, the three other substances externally travel through the yang of the lesser yang and internally travel through the yin of the terminal yin. Thus, the dredging and draining nature of the Liver and Gallbladder is satisfied and the terminal [yin] is unblocked.

This explanation, which places the Liver at the center, is completely in accordance with clinical reality.

PHYSICIAN A   The disease location for Frigid Extremities Powder *(sì nì sǎn)* is the Liver and yet in *Discussion of Cold Damage (Shāng hán lùn)*, the original line related to the formula (line 318) is placed in the lesser yin chapter: "A lesser yin disease with frigid extremities—the person may have coughing, or palpitations, or impeded urination, or pain in the abdomen, or diarrhea with down-bearing; Frigid Extremities Powder governs." Because this is obviously not a true lesser yin pattern, our textbook on the *Discussion of Cold Damage (Shāng hán lùn)* clearly explains:

> This line represents a mild pattern of heat inversion. Although, in the text, it is labeled as a lesser yin disease, it is different than the other lesser yin patterns of yang deficiency and yin abundance. It represents a pattern in which the qi dynamic is impeded, the yang qi is constrained in the interior and unable to thrust out to the exterior. In reality, this is owing to Liver and Stomach qi stagnation and yang constraint, resulting in mild inversion cold of the extremities.

However, the associated disease name, signs and symptoms, treatment method, and formula use seem disjointed. Generations of physicians have offered different explanations and been unable to agree. What is your view on this issue?

DR. YU   This issue is somewhat complicated. In reviewing the historical commentary on the Frigid Extremities Powder *(sì nì sǎn)* pattern, the explanations generally fall into one of three types.

The first type of explanation contends that Frigid Extremities Powder *(sì nì sǎn)* represents a deficiency-cold pattern. As the early 18th-century physician Qian Tian-Lai stated, "In lesser yin patients, as was stated previously [in line 281], the pulse is faint and fine, and there is a desire to just sleep." This explanation is directly derived from the source text, but it does not match with the functions or treatment actions of Frigid Extremities Powder *(sì nì sǎn)*. It is completely detached from clinical reality.

The second type of explanation posits that the Frigid Extremities Powder *(sì nì sǎn)* pattern represents a combined lesser yin and greater yin pattern. Thus, the treatment should be aimed at expelling yin, stopping diarrhea, tonifying the middle, and driving out thin mucus. Another 18th-century physician, Shu Chi-Yuan, wrote, "How should one use Frigid Extremities Powder *(sì nì sǎn)*? It is extremely difficult to understand [the use in this context.]" The notion is that Zhang Zhong-Jing made a mistake in choosing the formula or that later generations of writers misplaced some of the lines in the text. This perspective creates more problems than it solves.

The third type of explanation is that Frigid Extremities Powder *(sì nì sǎn)* represents a mild pattern of heat inversion. Further, that Frigid Extremities Powder *(sì nì sǎn)* is a fundamental formula for treating qi stagnation affecting the Liver and Stomach. This explanation is accepted by a clear majority of physicians and most modern physicians follow it.

PHYSICIAN C   However, it seems to me that no physicians, ancient or modern, have squarely addressed this issue. Lesser yin disease is characterized by Heart and Kidney deficiency; thus, the primary treatment method is to revive the yang and rescue from rebellion. The pathodynamic and treatment principle have nothing to do with Frigid Extremities Powder *(sì nì sǎn)*. And yet, Zhang Zhong-Jing not only placed this line in the lesser yin chapter, he starts the line off with the phrase "lesser yin disease," perhaps for fear that later generations would not know that this was a lesser yin disease. What is the meaning behind the seemingly mistaken placement of this line?

DR. YU   I believe that the placement of this line in the lesser yin chapter, although it seems to be a mistake, actually has import. Frigid Extremities Decoction *(sì nì tāng)* governs yang deficiency inversion counterflow occurring in lesser yin disease. Zhang Zhong-Jing placed the Frigid Extremities Powder *(sì nì sǎn)* pattern alongside this formula to avoid the situation where a physician, seeing counterflow cold of the extremities, assumes that it is the result of yang deficiency and yin abundance, and reflexively prescribes Frigid Extremities Decoction *(sì nì tāng)*. Between the two formula names, only one character is different, but that is intentional. We must be cautious because small discrepancies can lead to large errors!

To reiterate, counterflow cold of the extremities is not just observed in lesser yin disease. If upon seeing this symptom you immediately prescribe Frigid Extremities Decoction *(sì nì tāng)* to revive yang and rescue from rebellion, you will have gone far off track.

PHYSICIAN B If Zhang Zhong-Jing's intention was to aid differential diagnosis, why did he start the line with the phrase "lesser yin disease," which has confused countless generations of physicians?

DR. YU Although it is correct that the essence of the Frigid Extremities Powder *(sì nì sǎn)* pattern is not lesser yin, it is also true that it shares an important symptom, cold extremities, with lesser yin disease. Thus, we can view it as a lesser yin disease in terms of this symptom. In fact, there are other lines in the lesser yin chapter of *Discussion of Cold Damage (Shāng hán lùn)* aimed at aiding differential diagnosis. An example is line 324, which states, "For a lesser yin disease with vomiting right after ingesting food and drink, churning in the Heart with a desire to vomit but an inability to vomit again, if in the beginning of getting it the hands and feet are cold and the pulse wiry and slow, this is excess in the chest. It cannot be purged as vomiting should be used." In this line, one of the symptoms is cold extremities, which seems similar to lesser yin disease, yet the disease is not similar. This pattern is phlegm and food obstructing the chest and diaphragm. The obstruction causes an excess pattern of constrained yang and should be treated through inducing vomiting. Zhang Zhong-Jing begins the line with the phrase "lesser yin disease" because this pattern contains lesser yin disease manifestations. He created the theoretical system related to lesser yin disease, deeply revealed the true nature of the pattern as one of yang deficiency and yin abundance, and presented strict guidelines and standards for treatment. We can infer that, simultaneously, he was also using direct observation of the pattern manifestations of lesser yin disease to remind physicians of the absolute necessity of a deep engagement with the true nature of the illness, so as to avoid acting rashly when prescribing. As he decries in the preface to the text about the rash behavior of his contemporaries, "In reflecting on illnesses and inquiring of patients' suffering, their effort is placed on the gift of gab, and after a brief consultation, [they] give a simple prescription for a decoction."

PHYSICIAN A Do you have a textual basis for your understanding?

DR. YU Given the limitations of my own reading of the literature, to date, I have been unable to find textual support for my position. However, many of the commentators on *Discussion of Cold Damage (Shāng hán lùn)* that I most esteem seem to give quite strained interpretations of this issue that often seem disconnected from clinical reality. For example, Ke Yun-Bo reaches back to the *Inner Classic* and invokes the idea that "the lesser yin is the pivot." He then deduces that the pathodynamic of the Frigid Extremities Powder *(sì nì sǎn)* pattern is a loss of the governing function of the lesser yin pivot. Chen Xiu-Yuan echoes this idea and actually puts this in opposition to the idea of the lesser yang as the pivot: "The lesser yang is the yang pivot. Minor Bupleurum Decoction *(xiǎo chái hú tāng)* is a specialized formula for shifting the yang pivot. The lesser yin is the yin pivot. This powder (Frigid Extremities Powder *[sì nì sǎn]*) is a specialized formula for shifting the yin pivot." To me, this explanation is misusing the ideas of "the lesser yin is the pivot" and "the lesser yang is the pivot." This problem stems from confusing the basic nature of lesser yin disease with the outward appearance of the disease. As Karl Marx stated, "all science would be superfluous if the outward appearance and the essence of things directly coincided." Given this logic, when we consider the issue as it is discussed in modern textbooks on *Discussion of Cold Damage (Shāng hán lùn)*, the explanation of the Frigid Extremities Powder *(sì nì sǎn)* pattern as "similar to a lesser yang disease" or "a lesser yin disease concurrent with a lesser yang disease" is also quite unconvincing, because neither cold extremities nor diarrhea with tenesmus are typically present in lesser yang disease, whereas they are commonly seen in the Frigid Extremities Powder *(sì nì sǎn)* pattern.

My teacher, Jiang Er-Xun, who was a modern scholar of *Discussion of Cold Damage (Shāng hán lùn)*, believed that it made more sense to consider the Frigid Extremities Powder *(sì nì sǎn)* pattern a concurrent terminal yin pattern, rather than a concurrent lesser yang pattern. His rationale was that both cold extremities and diarrhea with tenesmus readily occur in terminal yin patterns. Furthermore, heat-type diarrhea with tenesmus is a special symptom associated with terminal yin patterns. Although Ke Yun-Bo sometimes used faulty logic in his analysis of the Frigid Extremities Powder *(sì nì sǎn)* pattern, he does place importance on the presence of diarrhea with tenesmus in the pattern. He suggests that this specific term should follow directly after cold extremities in line 318, and should not be considered a secondary symptom. Dr. Jiang spent his entire life reading and studying *Collected Writings on Renewal of the Discussion of Cold Damage (Shāng hán lái sū jí)* by Ke Yun-Bo. One day, as he was reading the section of the text related to Frigid Extremities Powder *(sì nì sǎn)*, he suddenly exclaimed, "This [text] is truly a rare find. What a pity that he only drilled down [into this issue] ninety percent; [his explanation] just leaves out the last ten percent."

CHAPTER 4

Pediatrics

4.1 Pediatric high fever

High fever for seven days

Breaking through fixed ideas

衝破思維定式

■ CASE HISTORY

Patient: *Chen, 10-year-old boy*

Seven days previously, the patient had developed chills and fever after swimming for too long and then getting repeatedly soaked by recent rain showers. He did not sweat but had generalized aches and weakness with a mild sore throat. His temperature was measured at 102.2°F (39°C).

He was initially given two packets of Honeysuckle and Forsythia Powder *(yín qiáo sǎn)* with Moslae Herba *(xiāng rú)* but this was ineffective. This was followed by an intramuscular injection of Bupleuri Radix *(chái hú)* and an andrographolide antibiotic along with orally administered acetaminophen, Six-Miracle Pill *(liù shén wán)* and Andrographitis Herba *(chuān xīn lián)*. The boy eventually broke a sweat and his fever abated, but several hours later his fever returned and he was brought into the emergency room and put under observation. Blood tests and a chest x-ray revealed nothing abnormal. The biomedical diagnosis was an "upper respiratory tract infection" and he was put on an IV drip containing primarily ampicillin and vitamins. Additionally, he was given antipyretic and analgesic medications. As before, his fever receded and then returned and at times reached 104.9°F

{63}

(40.5°C). Purple Snow Special Pill *(zǐ xuě dān)* was added in hopes of reducing his high fever, but this too was ineffective. All in all, the boy had experienced a high fever for about seven days, during which time he ate extremely little and gradually became thin and frail. After a consultation with the pediatricians at the hospital it was decided to give him steroids. The boy's parents, however, strenuously objected, and feeling very apprehensive, brought their son to see me.

INTAKE EXAMINATION
DATE: August 2, 1985

The patient lay supine on the clinic bed. His face was gaunt and his complexion dull, while his lips were red and dry. He didn't sweat much, had slight chills and his hands and feet were cold. His forehead and body, however, were hot and he also had a slight cough. He was generally listless but would occasionally become restless and unsettled. The boy had not had a bowel movement in three days and was thirsty and had the desire to drink. His throat was slightly red and his tongue was red with a thin, white, and slightly yellow coating that lacked moisture. The pulse was tight and rapid. His temperature was 103.1°F (39.5°C).

DIFFERENTIATION OF PATTERNS AND DISCUSSION OF TREATMENT

PHYSICIAN A   This patient had some very typical signs of febrile illness. In TCM textbooks the common cold *(gǎn mào)* is divided into three types: wind-heat, wind-cold, and summerheat pathogen. In this patient's case, the boy had a high fever that lasted seven days. Given the fact that he had become ill during the hottest time of summer, is it reasonable to assume that his condition was due to a summerheat pathogen and to treat him by clearing summerheat and releasing the exterior?

DR. YU   By definition a common cold due to a summerheat pathogen must be accompanied by dampness. In addition to damp-summerheat obstructing the protective yang qi and producing high fever, symptoms of damp-summerheat causing stagnation in the middle burner will also be prominent, such as stifling focal distention in the epigastrium or, in severe cases, vomiting and diarrhea. In this case there were no such symptoms, so for the time being we can rule out the possibility of damp-summerheat as a causative factor.

PHYSICIAN B   If the child's illness isn't due to a summerheat pathogen, then what type of pathogen can it be attributed to, wind-cold or wind-heat?

DR. YU   After seven days with a high fever, it is difficult to make a clear distinction between wind-cold and wind-heat. Objectively speaking, both the yin and yang of children's bodies are immature, as their bodies have not yet fully developed. Therefore, in children it is relatively rare that a common cold with high fever is due to either pure wind-cold or pure wind-heat. In most situations, the issue is one of external cold with internal heat, also known as 'cold enveloping heat.' This is the same as what the ancients called 'intruding cold enveloping fire.' There are differences between this and the high fever in adults with a common cold.

PHYSICIAN B   It seems that the symptoms of internal heat are quite obvious, but the external cold signs are not. How does the 'cold' in external cold with internal heat manifest?

DR. YU   Not being obvious doesn't mean the symptoms aren't there. The findings of mild chills, scant sweating, a thin, white tongue coating with a slight yellow tint, and a pulse that was somewhat tight are all indications of an external cold pathogen that hasn't resolved. In the clinic, it is important to pay close attention to whether there are signs of external cold. Just because a child has a high fever, don't disregard the possibility of external cold, and even more so, never use a thermometer to determine whether the illness is due to cold or heat.

PHYSICIAN C   You said that there are differences between adults and children with high fever due to common cold. Should I assume then that the treatments are different?

DR. YU   Yes, that's correct. In situations where common cold with high fever presents as cold enveloping heat then using a formula to strictly induce sweating and disperse cold with warm and acrid medicinal substances—for example, formulas such as Ephedra Decoction *(má huáng tāng)* or Schizonepeta and Saposhnikovia Powder to Overcome Pathogenic Influences *(jīng fáng bài dú sǎn)*—would be inappropriate. Even though the external cold pathogen may be eliminated, the internal heat will flare up. On the other hand, if strictly acrid and cool formulas that clear heat and release the exterior are used—such as Mulberry Leaf and Chrysanthemum Drink *(sāng jú yǐn)* and Honeysuckle and Forsythia Powder *(yín qiáo sǎn)*—then the exterior cold pathogen will linger and the internal heat won't have a pathway through which to escape.

My experience has shown that the most effective way to resolve the condition is to follow a method that uses acrid, warm medicinal substances paired with acrid, cool medicinal substances to unblock the pores and clear and vent accumulated heat as the primary method. This should be assisted by medicinal substances to turn the pivot and raise qi in order to guide the heat out. Additionally, further assistance by sour and sweet medicinal substances to generate yin, harmonize the nutritive qi and drain out heat, as well as strengthen the parts of the body that have not yet been affected, will be beneficial. Together these strategies will eliminate the illness in one fell swoop.

The pattern here is one of wind-cold entering the interior from the exterior and transforming into heat, which is a pattern of combined three yang disease. The treatment method is to disperse wind and cold, and clear and vent interior heat.

TREATMENT AND OUTCOME

FIRST VISIT: Bupleurum and Kudzu Decoction to Release the Muscle Layer *(chái gé jiě jī tāng)* completely follows these treatment strategies. It quickly reduces high fever due to common cold in children and is a steady and consistent formula. The child was given one packet of a modified Bupleurum and Kudzu Decoction to Release the Muscle Layer *(chái gé jiě jī tāng)*:

Bupleuri Radix *(chái hú)* 25g
Puerariae Radix *(gé gēn)* 30g
Angelicae dahuricae Radix *(bái zhǐ)* 10g

Notopterygii Rhizoma seu Radix *(qiāng huó)* 10g

Platycodi Radix *(jié gěng)* 10g

Glycyrrhizae Radix *(gān cǎo)* 5g

Paeoniae Radix alba *(bái sháo)* 10g

Scutellariae Radix *(huáng qín)* 6g

Gypsum fibrosum *(shí gāo)* 50g

Forsythiae Fructus *(lián qiào)* 10g

Uncariae Ramulus cum Uncis *(gōu téng)* 10g

Pheretima *(dì lóng)* 6g

Instructions: Take 500ml of water to precook the Gypsum fibrosum *(shí gāo)* for 30 minutes. Then add the remaining medicinal substances, except for Uncariae Ramulus cum Uncis *(gōu téng)*, and boil on a moderate heat for ten minutes. Finally, add the Uncariae Ramulus cum Uncis *(gōu téng)* and cook for three more minutes. After straining there should be about 300ml of decoction. The child should take 60ml of the decoction every half hour.

Results: After taking four doses the child began to perspire mildly over his entire body and his fever gradually abated. After completely finishing the decoction the child had a soft bowel movement, and his temperature was measured at 98.2°F (36.8°C). That night he slept peacefully without waking and the next morning his temperature was back to normal.

SECOND VISIT: Two packets of Lophatherum and Gypsum Decoction *(zhú yè shí gāo tāng)* were prescribed to consolidate the treatment. Afterwards the boy had no recurrence of fever. His parents were urged to make sure the child's diet was moderate in amount and balanced in flavor and temperature. The boy's health was gradually restored.

Disease	Primary symptoms	Differentiation	Treatment method	Formula
Common cold	High fever with mild chills, weariness with irritability and restlessness	External cold that hasn't been eliminated, and overabundance of internal heat	Disperse wind and cold, clear and vent interior heat	Bupleurum and Kudzu Decoction to Release the Muscle Layer *(chái gé jiě jī tāng)*

REFELCTIONS AND CLARIFICATIONS

PHYSICIAN A   The formula Bupleurum and Kudzu Decoction to Release the Muscle Layer *(chái gé jiě jī tāng)* was created by the Ming-dynasty physician Tao Hua and recorded in his book, *Six Texts on Cold Damage (Shāng hán liù shū)*. The formula consists of 11 herbs: Bupleuri Radix *(chái hú)*, Puerariae Radix *(gé gēn)*, Angelicae dahuricae Radix *(bái zhǐ)*, Notopterygii Rhizoma seu Radix *(qiāng huó)*, Gypsum fibrosum *(shí gāo)*, Platycodi Radix *(jié gěng)*, Scutellariae Radix *(huáng qín)*, Paeoniae Radix alba *(bái sháo)*, Glycyrrhizae Radix *(gān cǎo)*, Zingiberis Rhizoma recens *(shēng jiāng)*, and Jujubae Fructus *(dà zǎo)*. It was used as a substitute for Kudzu Decoction *(gé gēn tāng)* to treat combined *tái yáng* and *yáng míng* channel disease. Symptoms include diminishing chills with increasing generalized fever, headache, aching limbs, eye pain, dryness in the nose, irritability with insomnia, and distention and pain around the eyes.

Analyzing the herbs in the formula, it doesn't seem to completely match with the treatment methods you mentioned previously. However, you said that it does completely match. What is this assessment based on?

DR. YU   Historically, most of those who have sought to explain the construction of Bupleurum and Kudzu Decoction to Release the Muscle Layer *(chái gé jiě jī tāng)* have emphasized the nature, flavors and functions of each individual herb in the formula, rather than looking at it from the perspective of the combinations and synergy of herbs within the formula. My perspective is that the importance of this formula lies in the structure of herb pairs, and that Tao Hua ingeniously took the strategies of five different formulas, used the essence of each, and concentrated them down into these pairs to create a new formula. However, Tao Hua didn't reveal the formulas behind the combinations. He implied them but did not give specifics.

My own analysis of how it is constructed is as follows:

- Notopterygii Rhizoma seu Radix *(qiāng huó)* and Gypsum fibrosum *(shí gāo)*: An acrid, warm substance combined with an acrid, cold one. This is modeled after the treatment strategy of Major Bluegreen Dragon Decoction *(dà qīng lóng tāng)*: pushing wind-cold outward that has been bound to the exterior while clearing and venting excess heat that has accumulated internally.

- Puerariae Radix *(gé gēn)* and Angelicae dahuricae Radix *(bái zhǐ)*: This pair lightly clears heat while raising and dispersing. This pair is the essence of Cimicifuga and Kudzu Decoction *(shēng má gé gēn tāng)* and is excellent at releasing heat from the *yáng míng* muscle layer.

- Bupleuri Radix *(chái hú)* and Scutellariae Radix *(huáng qín)*: These are the primary herbs in Minor Bupleurum Decoction *(xiǎo chái hú tāng)*. This pair turns the pivot of *shǎo yáng* and leads pathogenic heat out of the body.

- Platycodi Radix *(jié gěng)* and Glycyrrhizae Radix *(gān cǎo)*: These two herbs comprise Platycodon and Licorice Decoction *(jié gěng gān cǎo tāng)*. This pair of herbs is light and clear and thus floats to the upper body to eliminate superficial heat from the chest, diaphragm, and throat.

- Paeoniae Radix alba *(bái sháo)* and Glycyrrhizae Radix *(gān cǎo)*: Together these two herbs comprise Peony and Licorice Decoction *(sháo yào gān cǎo tāng)*. The combination of sour and sweet flavors transforms yin, harmonizes nutritive qi, and discharges heat from constraint from the muscles and interstices.

Seen in its entirety, Bupleurum and Kudzu Decoction to Release the Muscle Layer *(chái gé jiě jī tāng)* contains the treatment strategies and essences of all the formulas mentioned above. Hence, the formula can simultaneously attend to externally-contracted pathogenic heat in all three diseased levels: exterior, interior, and half exterior/half interior. The formula disperses upward and outward, it clears and vents, and leads and guides pathogenic heat out of the body, leaving it nowhere to hide.

I understand, from repeated experience, that when using this formula, if the dosage, additions and cooking methods are all appropriate, it will be very effective in reducing high fever due to upper respiratory infection. In addition, the fever usually won't come back.

PHYSICIAN A   Can you please specify the dosages, additions, cooking method and method for taking the formula?

DR. YU   There are four herbs which must be included: Notopterygii Rhizoma seu Radix *(qiāng huó)*, Gypsum fibrosum *(shí gāo)*, Bupleuri Radix *(chái hú)*, and Puerariae Radix *(gé gēn)*. The dosages are Notopterygii Rhizoma seu Radix *(qiāng huó)* 3-10g, Gypsum fibrosum *(shí gāo)* 30g and above (the ratio between these two herbs must be between 1:5 and 1:10), the dosage of Bupleuri Radix *(chái hú)* should not be less than 25g, and Puerariae Radix *(gé gēn)* not less than 30g. The remaining herbs in the formula can be used according to their standard dosages.

Additions to the formula include the following:

- For particularly severe sore throat, add Belamcandae Rhizoma *(shè gān)* 6g and Lasiosphaera/Calvatia *(mǎ bó)* 10g.
- If summerheat is part of the pattern, add 10g of Moslae Herba *(xiāng rú)* and 15g of Talcum *(huá shí)*.
- If food stagnation is present, add dry-fried Raphani Semen *(lái fú zǐ)*, 10g.
- If fright (wind) is part of the pattern, add 10g each of Uncariae Ramulus cum Uncis *(gōu téng)* and Pheretima *(dì lóng)*.

Even though the boy didn't show any signs of fright wind pattern with spasms or convulsions, given that he had a high fever for seven days, at one time reaching 104.9°F (40.5°C), this combination was used in his formula to prevent fright collapse.

Cooking method: Gypsum fibrosum *(shí gāo)* should be pre-cooked for 30 minutes. The remaining ingredients should be boiled on high heat for ten minutes. The herbs should only be decocted once.

It is challenging to give Chinese medicine to children. If the standard method of taking decoctions three times per day is followed, it is difficult for the child to take enough and the time between doses is too long. This will lengthen the time it takes to reduce the child's fever. When I first started using this formula, I struggled with the issue of the best way for the patient to take the medicine. Eventually I discovered that it was best to have children take the medicine more frequently and in small doses. This made it easier for children to accept, as well as making the overall intake adequate and the effects continuous.

    Observation of many patients has shown that, in most cases, about two hours after taking the first dose the child will begin to sweat mildly, and the fever will start to gradually recede. After finishing one to two packets of medicine, when the patient's temperature has returned to normal, I consolidate the treatment by turning to Lophatherum and Gypsum Decoction *(zhú yè shí gāo tāng)*. This boosts qi, engenders fluids, and continues to clear any remnants of heat in the body.

PHYSICIAN B   I'd like to ask another question. Since the child, at one point, hadn't had a bowel movement for three days, could you not also have considered using purgatives?

DR. YU   Although the child hadn't had a bowel movement for three days, he didn't have any signs of bowel fullness such as abdominal bloating or abdominal pain that worsens with pressure. How could purgatives be appropriate?

PHYSICIAN B   Here we have a child with a high fever lasting for seven days, and despite the continuous use of numerous Chinese and Western medicines, his fever still came back again and again. The doctors were seemingly out of options, it's no wonder they wanted to use steroids, their trump card. In terms of his initial treatment, were there really no other options? I think this is truly worth reexamining!

DR. YU   You are absolutely correct. It seems that there is a trend among some doctors when treating high fever due to the common cold to avoid using acrid, warm medicinal substances at all costs and consider Mulberry Leaf and Chrysanthemum Drink *(sāng jú yǐn)* and Honeysuckle and Forsythia Powder *(yín qiáo sǎn)* to be as valuable as gold. Then there is another type of doctor. This type immediately begins their treatment by prescribing antipyretics or antibiotics for any patient with a high fever without careful consideration of the cause of the illness, its pathodynamics, or the constitution of the patient. Then, as a back-up, they follow this with cold, bitter medicinal substances such as Lonicerae Flos *(jīn yín huā)*, Isatidis/Baphicacanthis Radix *(bǎn lán gēn)* and Isatidis Folium *(dà qīng yè)*, or negligently prescribe highly sweetened 'instant granules.' A few days will pass and if the fever doesn't go down, the family becomes anxious and the doctor becomes confused as to what to do. Formulas that are meant to treat heat in the nutritive and blood aspects, such as Purple Snow Special Pill *(zǐ xuě dān)*, Greatest Treasure Special Pill *(zhì bǎo dān)* and Calm the Palace Pill with Cattle Gallstone *(ān gōng niú huáng wán)*, are boldly brought out as a defense. Then there are those doctors who will resort to steroids. These medical 'conventions' have been taught to many and the results have been extremely detrimental. We urgently need a program to change old conventions and habits.

4.2 Pediatric night sweats

Child with night sweats for two years

Children are not miniature adults

小兒不是成人的縮影

■ CASE HISTORY

Patient: *Ms. Zhang, 5-year-old girl*

The patient has suffered from night sweats for the past two years. She has low-grade fevers at night and once she falls asleep she sweats over her entire body. The sweating stops as soon as she awakes. Her sweat is cold and sticky. Occasionally the child will sweat so much that her undergarments become soaked.

INTAKE EXAMINATION
DATE: September 15, 1985

Observation: The child was fatigued and sleepy. She was underweight, her complexion was pale and dusky and the pupils of her eyes had a greenish tinge.

She had a dry mouth and liked to drink, her food intake was poor, and her stools dry. Her tongue was pale red with a thin, white coating that lacked moisture. Her pulse was wiry and moderate.

An x-ray of her lungs showed no abnormalities. Biomedical doctors considered this to be a case of poor nutrition and a zinc deficiency. However, despite prolonged treatment there was no improvement.

Previously the patient had intermittently taken more than 20 packets of Tangkuei and Six-Yellow Decoction *(dāng guī liù huáng tāng)* and Anemarrhena, Phellodendron, and Rehmannia Pill *(zhī bǎi dì huáng wán)* along with medicinal substances that anchor yang and have suppressing and containing functions. At this point the child's parents had already lost hope that their child's health would improve. They had heard that members of the "Master Students Group of Jiang Er-Xun" had opened a clinic specializing in difficult disorders, so they made a special trip to our clinic in Leshan to see if we could help.

DIFFERENTIATION OF PATTERNS AND DISCUSSION OF TREATMENT

PHYSICIAN A   Textbooks say that night sweats (盗汗 *dào hàn*) are due to yin deficiency. This is logical because night is associated with yin, and if someone sweats during the night, it must be the result of yin deficiency. On the other hand, there are patients who sweat incessantly when they nap during the daytime. Is this also because of yin deficiency?

DR. YU   First, we should clarify the definition of *dào hàn* (generally translated as night sweats). Regardless of whether it's during the night or during the day, if sweating begins upon entering sleep and stops upon waking, this is called *dào hàn*. As Zhu Dan-Xi said in his book *Essential Teachings of [Zhu] Dan-Xi (Dān-Xī xīn fǎ)*, "A person with night sweats is described as having sweating that begins when [they] enter asleep, and if they don't sleep, sweat will not issue forth. Only when they are sleeping deeply [does the sweat] pour forth, when they awaken [it] stops and doesn't come out again. This is unlike the spontaneous excretion [of sweat] that occurs in spontaneous sweating." This is the concept of night sweats *(dào hàn)*.[1]

In the *Indispensable Tools for Pattern Treatment (Zhèng zhì zhǔn shéng)* the cause and pathodynamic of *dào hàn* can be summarized as various disease factors that have "damaged and harmed yin-blood and enfeebled the qi of the form. When yin qi is deficient, it cannot pair with yang. Thus, internally, yang qi steams and manifests externally as night sweats." So, it doesn't matter whether it is during the nighttime or the daytime,

---

1. A literal translation of the term 盗汗 *dào hàn* would be 'thieving sweats.' The genesis of this term is probably due to this type of sweating occurring when the person is unaware of it (i.e., sleeping) and thus is analogous to a thief taking advantage of someone's inattention to steal valuables. The valuables here are the patient's yin and fluids.

sleep belongs to yin and when yin is deficient, yang flares. As it says in Chapter 7 of the *Basic Questions*, "Yang added into yin is called sweat."

In terms of patterns seen in the clinic, night sweats associated with an externally-contracted disease is usually due to pathogens attached to *shào yáng*, while most night sweats from the miscellaneous illnesses or internal damage are attributed to yin deficiency. Night sweats due to qi deficiency, yang deficiency, or damp-heat are relatively uncommon.

PHYSICIAN A   The majority of ancient and modern medical texts have clearly ascribed the cause of night sweats to yin-deficiency internal heat with yang losing the ability to anchor and store. The standard treatment method is to enrich yin and direct fire downward, and anchor yang while suppressing and containing. Why is it that in this case, the child was given formulas that have all of these functions and yet nothing worked?

DR. YU   Tangkuei and Six-Yellow Decoction *(dāng guī liù huáng tāng)* and Anemarrhena, Phellodendron, and Rehmannia Pill *(zhī bǎi dì huáng wán)* have an abundance of cold and cool herbs to direct fire downward but are insufficient in herbs that enrich the Spleen and restrain the Liver. These formulas are useful for adults but are not very apt for children who present with a weak Spleen and an exuberant Liver.

The concern is that these formulas, when given to a child, will likely damage the Spleen and weaken the Stomach. This is particularly common when practitioners prescribe these formulas and, after seeing no improvement after two or three packets, prescribe a few more because they are operating under the illusion that the herbs haven't yet taken effect.

In the present case, even though the child was feverish during the night and had night sweats, none of the other symptoms indicated any signs of internal heat or exuberant fire; not the pale red tongue, the thin, white coating that lacked moisture, nor the wiry, moderate pulse. Moreover, it was clear that the formulas the girl took didn't improve her situation.

Based on the child's symptoms, pulse, and tongue the diagnosis was clear: Spleen yin exhaustion with Liver exuberance and floating yang. The strategy was to enrich the Spleen and restrain the Liver, and anchor and contain floating yang. I prescribed a modification of Zhang Xi-Chun's Decoction to Sustain Life *(zī shēng tāng)*. Six packets were given:

Dioscoreae Rhizoma *(shān yào)*	30g
Scrophulariae Radix *(xuán shēn)*	15g
Atractylodis macrocephalae Rhizoma *(bái zhú)*	10g
Gigeriae galli Endothelium corneum *(jī nèi jīn)*	6g
Arctii Fructus *(niú bàng zǐ)*	[dry-fried and crushed] 6g
Paeoniae Radix alba *(bái sháo)*	10g
Fossilia Ossis Mastodi *(lóng gǔ)*	30g
Ostreae Concha *(mǔ lì)*	30g
Lycii Cortex *(dì gǔ pí)*	10g

SECOND VISIT: September 27

Result: After two packets of the formula the patient's nighttime feverishness and night sweats had significantly diminished; these symptoms had gradually come to an end by the time she finished the sixth packet. In addition, her appetite had begun to improve, she no longer had a dry mouth, and her bowel movements were smooth. She had a pale red tongue with a thin, white coating and a moderate pulse.

FORMULA:

> Dioscoreae Rhizoma *(shān yào)* 900g
> Gigeriae galli Endothelium corneum *(jī nèi jīn)* 30g

Instructions: Grind the herbs into a fine powder. Each morning cook 30g of the powder into a porridge and add sugar to taste. Continue to do this every day for one month.

Six months later the family was contacted and they reported no recurrence of symptoms. They also said that the child's complexion had returned to normal and the greenish tinge to the pupils of her eyes was gone.

Disease	Primary symptoms	Differential diagnosis	Treatment method	Formula
Night sweats	Night sweats, low grade fever	Spleen yin depletion with Liver exuberance and floating yang	Enrich the Spleen and restrain the Liver, anchor and contain floating yang	Zhang Xi-Chun's Decoction to Sustain Life *(zī shēng tāng)*

REFLECTIONS AND CLARIFICATIONS

PHYSICIAN D   In this case you mention a greenish tinge to the patient's pupils. This is not something that we have observed. How can pupils be green and what is the significance of this finding?

DR. YU   With malnourishment, children with a weakened Spleen and an exuberant Liver can also have depleted Kidney essence. As the water cannot restrain wood, the color of the wood will appear and the pupils will have a greenish tinge instead of being pure black. As these pathologies resolve, the unusual color will disappear. Nowadays, with malnutrition being very rare in China, this finding is also quite rare.

PHYSICIAN B   Spleen weakness and Liver exuberance is a general pathology for various illnesses in children, and not really specific enough to describe the pathology of night sweats. Yet a modification of Decoction to Sustain Life *(zī shēng tāng)*, designed to enrich the Spleen, restrain the Liver, and anchor and contain floating yang, was quite effective. What's the logic behind this?

DR. YU   Generalities exist within particularities. No doubt the symptom of night sweats is due to yin exhaustion and depletion of fluids, and yang losing its ability to anchor and store. But where is the source of this loss of balance between yin and yang? Apart from the symptoms of night fever and night sweats, the symptoms of weariness, sleepiness, loss of weight, pale, dusky complexion, a tinge of green color in the iris of the eyes, dry mouth with a desire to drink, a poor appetite and dry stools, can all be explained by four words: 'Spleen weakness' and 'Liver exuberance.'

More concretely, the term Spleen weakness refers to insufficient Spleen yin. If Spleen yin is insufficient, the ability to create yin essence is diminished and this leads to physical exhaustion. As for the term Liver exuberance, we can define this more specifically and say that it refers to inadequate Liver yin and the relative exuberance of the ministerial fire stored within the Liver. When the Liver is exuberant, not only will it encroach upon the Spleen, but the chances of it consuming yin essence increases as well.

This is the underlying cause of the patient's physical exhaustion, nighttime feverishness, and night sweats. The more physically exhausted the patient, the worse their nighttime feverishness and sweating become. The opposite is also true (the worse the feverishness and sweating, the more exhausted the patient becomes) and thus a vicious cycle develops. To stop this vicious cycle, the primary aspect of treatment must be to enrich the Spleen and restrain the Liver. When the root is approached this way, good results occur spontaneously.

PHYSICIAN C   There are numerous formulas that meet the requirements for enriching the Spleen and restraining the Liver, why choose Decoction to Sustain Life *(zī shēng tāng)?*

DR. YU   Decoction to Sustain Life *(zī shēng tāng)* was Zhang Xi-Chun's principal formula for treating yin deficiency consumption-heat. It was recorded in the first volume of his book, *Essays on Medicine Esteeming the Chinese Respecting the Western (Yī xué zhōng zhōng cān xī lù).* I have always been of the mind that this formula's primary function is to enrich Spleen yin.

Dioscoreae Rhizoma *(shān yào)*, in a large dosage, greatly enriches Spleen yin. It also assists Atractylodis macrocephalae Rhizoma *(bái zhú)* in strengthening the transporting function of the Spleen qi (Spleen qi deficiency usually accompanies Spleen yin deficiency, so simultaneous tonification is beneficial). As an assistant, Gigeriae galli Endothelium corneum *(jī nèi jīn)* is used not only for its ability to dissipate food stagnation and grind down accumulations, but more importantly because Gigeriae galli Endothelium corneum *(jī nèi jīn)* (which is the Spleen-Stomach of chickens) tonifies and nourishes the Spleen and Stomach in a 'like-treats-like' manner. Scrophulariae Radix *(xuán shēn)* is used to reduce deficiency heat, while Arctii Fructus *(niú bàng zǐ)* moistens the Lung and lubricates the intestines to unblock the bowels.

I add Paeoniae Radix alba *(bái sháo)* to the original formula to restrain the Liver, Moutan Cortex *(mǔ dān pí)* and Lycii Cortex *(dì gǔ pí)* to help Scrophulariae Radix *(xuán shēn)* reduce deficiency heat, and Fossilia Ossis Mastodi *(lóng gǔ)* and Ostreae Concha *(mǔ lì)* to anchor and contain floating yang.

PHYSICIAN C   Was Spleen yin one of the patterns that premodern physicians considered when treating night sweats?

DR. YU   Yes. One example is the Qing-dynasty physician Chen Xiu-Yuan. He liked to use Nelumbo, Jujube and Wild Soybean Decoction *(lián zǎo mǎ dòu tāng)* for treating night sweats. Nelumbinis Semen *(lián zǐ)*, Jujubae Fructus *(dà zǎo)* and Glycine soja *(mǎ liào dòu)* are herbs that enrich Spleen yin.

A further example is another Qing-dynasty physician, Lin Pei-Qin, who liked to use Augment the Yin Decoction *(yì yīn tāng)* for night sweats. This formula is based on the yin-enriching formula Six-Ingredient Pill with Rehmannia *(liù wèi dì huáng wán)*. It also contains Ophiopogonis Radix *(mài mén dōng)* and Nelumbinis Semen *(lián zǐ)* to enrich Spleen yin, Paeoniae Radix alba *(bái sháo)* and Schisandrae Fructus *(wǔ wèi zǐ)* to restrain the Liver, Lycii Cortex *(dì gǔ pí)* to reduce deficiency heat, and Junci Medulla *(dēng xīn cǎo)* to guide heat downward.

I have done some testing of these formulas in my practice and neither of them is as effective as this modification of Decoction to Sustain Life *(zī shēng tāng)*.

PHYSICIAN D   Is there much opportunity in the clinic to use this modified version of Decoction to Sustain Life *(zī shēng tāng)*?

DR. YU   Many, many opportunities. I almost always use a modification of this formula when treating night sweats in children. This is something I am very familiar with and I have used the formula again and again. It has never let me down.

There is a country doctor, surname is Zhu, who tells a story of his eight-year-old child who suffered from night sweats for two months. Dr. Zhu gave the child a formula to enrich yin and anchor yang, but it was ineffective. He came to me specifically looking for a formula, so I showed him this formula with some additions. He looked at it and an expression came over his face as if he couldn't believe what he saw. I said to him, "Try two packets of this, it can't do any harm." Not long after he came back to tell me, "Sure enough, all it took was two packets and the night sweats just stopped!"

If after taking several packets of this formula your patient's night sweats have improved but not completely stopped, you can add 30g of Agrimoniae Herba *(xiān hè cǎo)*. If the patient has night sweats as well as spontaneous sweating, you can add 15-30g of Astragali Radix *(huáng qí)* to the formula.

PHYSICIAN B   In this patient's case, her night sweats had resolved, but you gave her Dioscoreae Rhizoma *(shān yào)* and Gigeriae galli Endothelium corneum *(jī nèi jīn)* as food therapy for a month longer. Is this necessary?

DR. YU   Very necessary. The reason is that even though the night sweats had recently resolved, the root of the illness, the patient's Spleen yin insufficiency, was still present. It's imperative then to continue to enrich Spleen yin and replenish the 'source of regeneration' to ensure there won't be a recurrence of the condition.

Dioscoreae Rhizoma *(shān yào)* is a common food product in China. Its flavor is sweet, which is the flavor associated with the Spleen, and so it can greatly enrich Spleen yin. Its color is white and thus it enters the Lung, and its juice is viscous, so it enters the Kidneys. Hence Dioscoreae Rhizoma *(shān yào)* both moistens the Lung and enriches the Kidneys.

A small dose of Gigeriae galli Endothelium corneum *(jī nèi jīn)* dissipates and guides out; it acts as an assistant to transport and transform the tonifying strength of Dioscoreae Rhizoma *(shān yào)* thus helping to avoid the stifling distention that might come from eating this porridge over a prolonged period. Adding sugar makes it tastier and will insure that children will definitely like it.

Zhang Xi-Chun often used this approach to consolidate the treatment for various types of illness where the patient had depleted yin and qi. It is worth learning from his experience. Master Zhang's approach to using Dioscoreae Rhizoma *(shān yào)* porridge derives from four words in Chapter 70 of the *Basic Questions (Sù wèn)*: "Finish with food nourishment." This is, without a doubt, a very effective path to recuperation.

4.3 Pediatric food aversion

Child averse to food for four months

A condition that has yet to garner sufficient clinical atttention

尚未引起臨證者足夠重視

■ CASE HISTORY

Patient: *5-year-old boy*

The child's mother reported that since her child was three-years old she had been giving him cod liver oil and various enriching tonics and supplements, that he often ate snacks, and that his appetite had been in a gradual decline. In the past four months, the child has begun to dislike food and at times would refuse to eat at all. Force feeding would result in screaming and retching.

One of their previous doctors told the mother to stop giving the child fish liver oil, all supplements, and to cut down on the boy's snacking. The doctor prescribed Crataegi Fructus *(shān zhā)* granules and Preserve Harmony Decoction *(bǎo hé tāng)* for seven days. This helped the child's appetite somewhat, but after eating he would often retch.

Subsequently, another doctor gave the child a decoction of Seven-Ingredient Powder with White Atractylodes *(qī wèi bái zhú sǎn)* and a decoction of Pill to Sustain Life and Strengthen the Spleen *(zī sheng jiàn pǐ wán)*, with instructions to take them alternately for seven to eight days. Nevertheless, at the end of a week the child still experienced an aversion to food.

Intake Examination
Date: December 5, 1993

The child was underweight and his complexion was slightly yellow and a bit dusky. His pupils had a green tint. The mother said that the child was quick to anger, slept poorly, was often thirsty, and had dry stools.

The boy's tongue was slightly red with a thin, yellow coating that lacked moisture. His pulse was wiry and fine.

Differentiation of Patterns and Discussion of Treatment

PHYSICIAN A   Food aversion is a term currently used in Chinese medicine, but there seems to be no such term in the ancient literature. Modern Chinese pediatric medicine textbooks say that food aversion refers to a common disorder in children. Over a relatively long period of time children with food aversion lack any strong desire for food, have a reduced appetite, or, in extreme cases, refuse to eat. The textbooks explain that the primary pathodynamic of this disorder is disharmony between the Spleen and Stomach that results in reduced food intake and loss of the transporting and transforming functions of the Spleen. Consequently, the focus of treatment is on the Spleen and Stomach. Medicated Leaven, Barley Sprout, Unripe Bitter Orange, and Atractylodes Pill *(qū mài zhǐ zhú wán)* is recommended for cases where the Spleen has lost its ability to transport food, Nourish the Stomach and Increase the Fluids Decoction *(yǎng wèi zēng yè tāng)*[2] for cases of Stomach yin insufficiency, and Ginseng, Poria, and White Atractylodes Powder *(shēn líng bái zhú sǎn)* for children with signs of Spleen and Stomach qi deficiency.

In your opinion what was the reason that the previous doctor's treatment of Spleen and Stomach was ineffective?

DR. YU   In recent years, along with the gradual material improvements in the lives of the average Chinese, the occurrence of children suffering from food aversion has increased. There are some patients who have taken formulas that either disperse food and open the Stomach, fortify the Spleen and augment qi, or nourish Stomach yin, and get no relief. This has been a source of consternation for many doctors. As the saying goes, extreme difficulties lead to changes in thinking. Zhang Zhong-Jing wrote that, "When seeing Liver disease, know that Liver [disorders] will be transmitted to the Spleen, so first bolster the Spleen." This is a concrete lesson of the principle of mutual control within the five phases. The principle of mutual control means that "I control you and you control me." So, I asked myself, is it possible to deduce from this idea that the opposite may also be true?

PHYSICIAN A   If we flip this idea around and assume the converse is true, it would give us: "When seeing Spleen disease, know that Spleen [problems] will be transmitted to the Liver, so first nourish the Liver."

DR. YU   Exactly! We have tried various methodologies including nourishing the Liver, soothing the Liver, and restraining the Liver to treat this condition and found that treatment outcomes were greatly improved when using these treatment principles. This goes to show that there is a strong relationship between food aversion and an exuberant Liver.

If, in addition to food aversion, the patient is underweight, has a dusky complexion, suffers from restless sleep, is easily angered or frightened, and has dry stools, this is more reason to treat the Liver as the primary source of pathology. The case here is just such an example.

It was our determination that the pattern in this child's case was one of Liver exuberance with Spleen weakness and a Stomach that had lost its moisture and its ability to direct rebellion downwards. We determined that treatment should focus on soothing the Liver, supporting the Spleen, nourishing the Stomach and directing rebellious qi downward. I prescribed my formula Soothe the Liver and Enrich the Stomach Decoction *(shū gān zī wèi tāng)*.

....

2. This is a modern formula developed by the authors of a pediatrics textbook. It consists of Dendrobii Herba *(shí hú)*, Mume Fructus *(wū méi)*, Glehniae Radix *(běi shā shēn)*, Polygonati odorati Rhizoma *(yù zhú)*, Paeoniae Radix alba *(bái sháo)*, and Glycyrrhizae Radix *(gān cǎo)*.

Treatment and Outcome

First visit: Two packets of Soothe the Liver and Enrich the Stomach Decoction *(shū gān zī wèi tāng)* were given:

Bupleuri Radix *(chái hú)* 10g
Scutellariae Radix *(huáng qín)* 6g
Trichosanthis Radix *(tiān huā fěn)* 10g
Paeoniae Radix alba *(bái sháo)* 12g
dry-fried Aurantii Fructus immaturus *(chǎo zhǐ shí)* 10g
Mume Fructus *(wū méi)* 10g
Polygoni cuspidati Rhizoma *(hǔ zhàng)* 12g
Coptidis Rhizoma *(huáng lián)* 3g
Forsythiae Fructus *(lián qiào)* 10g
Glehniae Radix *(běi shā shēn)* 12g
Saccharum cristallisatum *(bīng táng)* . . . . [rock sugar] 15g

Instructions: Soak the herbs in cold water for one hour. Cook on a low boil for 30 minutes. Drain and keep the strained decoction. Add water and repeat cooking for 30 minutes. Again, strain the decoction and mix the two strained decoctions together for a total of approximately 150ml. Divide into five doses taken warm throughout the day.

Additionally, make a tea from 30g each of roasted Cassiae Semen *(jué míng zǐ)* and rock sugar by steeping them together in hot water. Have the child drink some of this tea whenever he is thirsty. I also recommended that the child eliminate snacking.

Second visit: After starting the herbs the child was no longer retching. He also said he enjoyed drinking the Cassiae Semen *(jué míng zǐ)* and sugar tea. By the time he had finished the two packets of herbs he had passed dry stools three times, and his mother was able to coerce him into eating a small amount of food. His sleep improved slightly.

As I've said before, we should not change the basic formula when it is effective. Twelve grams of both Lilii Bulbus *(bǎi hé)* and Raphani Semen *(lái fú zǐ)* were added to the formula, and the boy was given two more packets. The patient continued with the Cassiae Semen *(jué míng zǐ)* and rock sugar tea.

Herbal porridge recipe:

Pseudostellariae Radix *(tài zǐ shēn)* 30g
Dioscoreae Rhizoma *(shān yào)* 30g
Poria *(fú líng)* 15g
Glycyrrhizae Radix praeparata *(zhì gān cǎo)* 5g
Lablab Semen album *(bái biǎn dòu)* 15g
Lilii Bulbul *(bǎi hé)* 20g
Nelumbinis Semen *(lián zǐ)* (remove the plumule) 20g
Glehniae Radix *(běi shā shēn)* 30g
Nonglutinous rice *(jīng mǐ)* 500g

Instructions: Roast the herbs until crisp and grind into a very fine powder. Dry-fry the Nonglutinous rice *(jīng mǐ)* until its cooked through. Grind into a fine powder and mix together with the herbs.

Take 20g of the powdered mixture and cook with an appropriate amount of water to make porridge. White sugar can be added to taste. Eat this porridge twice a day, morning and evening, before meals.

RESULT: After finishing roughly half of the herbal porridge, the child began to feel hungry and ask for food. His stools were regular, his sleep had improved, and his complexion also gradually improved.

Condition	Primary symptoms	Pattern differentiation	Treatment method	Formula
Aversion to food	Aversion to food, quick to anger, constipation, poor sleep	Liver exuberance and Spleen weakness, lack of moisture in the Stomach affecting its descending function	Soothe the Liver, support the Spleen, enrich the Stomach and direct rebellious qi downward	Soothe the Liver and Enrich the Stomach Decoction (shū gān zī wèi tāng)

REFLECTIONS AND CLARIFICATIONS

PHYSICIAN A   Dr. Yu, would you please explain in more detail why this formula, Soothe the Liver and Enrich the Stomach Decoction *(shū gān zī wèi tāng)*, is so effective in treating this type of food aversion?

DR. YU   This formula is a combination of Minor Bupleurum Decoction *(xiǎo chái hú tāng)* and Frigid Extremities Powder *(sì nì sǎn)* from the *Discussion of Cold Damage (Shāng hán lùn)*, and Coptis and Mume Decoction *(lián méi tang)* from the *Systematic Differentiation of Warm Pathogen Diseases (Wēn bìng tiáo biàn)*. It relies on the combination of acrid and bitter herbs and sour and sweet herbs. The acrid flavor disperses the Liver while the bitter flavor drains Heart fire (when there is excess, drain the child). Sour restrains Liver yin while sweet nourishes Stomach yin. Hence, as a whole, the formula soothes the Liver, supports the Spleen, enriches the Stomach and directs rebellious qi downward. Combining the treatment with Cassiae Semen *(jué míng zǐ)* and rock sugar tea serves to further enrich the Stomach, moisten the Intestines, and unblock the bowels. Once the Intestines were unblocked, the Stomach qi could immediately descend, and the child's appetite increased. This combination of Soothe the Liver and Enrich the Stomach Decoction *(shū gān zī wèi tāng)* with Cassiae Semen *(jué míng zǐ)* and rock sugar tea brings rapid results.

Reflecting upon my past treatment of this condition, I had believed everything in books and had concentrated on treating the Spleen and Stomach, but the results were poor. I pondered long and hard over what the converse theory would be. Surprisingly, I had forgotten Zhu Dan-Xi's famous words where he pointed out that, in children, the "Liver is frequently over-abundant."

PHYSICIAN B   Chinese medicine textbooks affirm that the Liver frequently being over-abundant is an important pathodynamic in children. However, in those textbooks the idea of the Liver frequently being over-abundant refers to the tendency of children to develop symptoms of high fever or convulsions when they are ill. In other words, this phrase about the Liver and over-abundance is a way of saying that children commonly develop signs that are due to stirring of Liver wind.

It seems, however, that you mean something else when you say that the Liver is frequently over-abundant; that you are referring to the emotional aspect as a cause. I'm afraid it would be difficult for most doctors to accept this new viewpoint of yours. People will question whether there really is a connection between the emotions and illnesses in children as young as four or five years old.

DR. YU Of course there is a connection! But I must say, the situation is not the same as it is in adults. Children's bodies are in a state of immature yin and immature yang. This means that their organs are delicate, and their bodies and brains are not fully developed, therefore disorders in children that are brought on by the seven emotions differ from emotionally-caused disorders in adults. On the one hand, children aren't necessarily as vulnerable as adults to emotions such as worry, excessive thinking, and grief. There is a line from an ancient poem that goes, "When young I never knew the taste of sorrow."[3] Yes, there are those rare children who have the talent to recite or write poetry, but their works tend to be contrived, as implied by the above poem, which continues, "For to compose new verses, I strained to speak of sorrow."

On the other hand, children are much more inclined to emotions and feelings such as anger, shock, and fear. It is not uncommon for children to become ill after experiencing these feelings intensely. This is particularly true of only children whose parents spoil them and who develop bad tempers. They can become willful or act out, and are often referred to as 'little emperors' here in China. These behaviors are manifestations of Liver exuberance. These 'little emperors' love to eat junk food, are often picky eaters, or refuse to eat any food that doesn't suit their tastes. Over time their appetites suffer, and they eventually develop an aversion to food.

The brilliant early-Qing doctor Ye Tian-Shi said, "The Liver is the source from which disease arises; the Stomach is where disease is transmitted." While this wasn't originally referring to the symptom of food aversion, is it not an apt description of the pathodynamic of food aversion in children? Because of the emotional component of this condition, treatment of symptoms should not be limited to medicinal substances, but rather combining herbal medicine with teaching the child good eating habits. As for methodology, if the focus of treatment isn't directed at the Liver, then the treatment will be in vain.

Currently many scholars are very focused on the various transformations between different medical models. For example, models that were once considered to be simply biological are being transformed into a biological-social-psychological model, which emphasizes the importance of the psychosomatic aspect of illness. My impression is that these models seem to be completely focused on adults, and don't include children. It's very unfortunate that the relationship between childhood illnesses and emotional factors hasn't garnered sufficient clinical attention.

PHYSICIAN C In this instance of food aversion, the pathodynamic was Liver exuberance, Spleen deficiency, and Stomach yin deficiency. The experiential formula you created and prescribed was effective because it addressed that pattern. What formula would you prescribe when presented with Liver exuberance and Spleen deficiency that does not include a dry mouth and dry stools or other signs of Stomach yin damage?

....
3. This is the beginning of a poem by the Southern Song patriot, Xin Qi-Ji 辛棄疾, probably written in the late 12th century.

__DR. YU__　A modified Zanthoxyli and Mume Decoction *(jiāo méi tang)* from the *Systematic Differentiation of Warm Pathogen Diseases (Wēn bìng tiáo biàn)* would be useful:

Mume Fructus *(wū méi)*.. 10g
Pseudostellariae Radix *(tài zǐ shēn)* 10g
Paeoniae Radix alba *(bái sháo)*................................... 10g
Dioscoreae Rhizoma *(shān yào)* 10g
Coptidis Rhizoma *(huáng lián)*.................................... 1.5g
Zingiberis Rhizoma *(gān jiāng)*.................................... 1.5g
Pinelliae Rhizoma praeparatum *(zhì bàn xià)* 6g
dry-fried Aurantii Fructus *(chǎo zhǐ ké)* 6g
Gigeriae galli Endothelium corneum *(jī nèi jīn)* 6g
Coptidis Rhizoma *(huáng lián)*.................................... 3g

This formula drains the *jué yīn*, harmonizes the *shào yáng*, and protects the *yáng míng*. It is remarkably effective for opening the Stomach and increasing the appetite. In most cases, the patient's appetite will show signs of improvement after two or three packets of this formula. I usually follow this formula with Seven-Ingredient Powder with White Atractylodes *(qī wèi bái zhú sǎn)* with the addition of Paeoniae Radix alba *(bái sháo)*, Mume Fructus *(wū méi)* and Gigeriae galli Endothelium corneum *(jī nèi jīn)* to carefully complete the treatment.

__PHYSICIAN C__　There are some cases of food aversion where it seems certain that the location of the pathology is limited to the Spleen and Stomach, that is, where there are no signs of Liver channel involvement. Nonetheless, formulas and herbs that disperse and guide, fortify, and assist transport are ineffective. What is the best treatment for those cases?

__DR. YU__　It is important to distinguish whether or not the condition is one of dual deficiency of qi and yin in the Spleen and Stomach. This would be the diagnosis if, in addition to food aversion, one sees symptoms of fatigue and weakness, tendency to sweat, mouth and lips that lack moisture, stools that are sometimes dry and sometimes loose, and a pale tongue with scant yang fluids. In such cases it is important to prescribe substances that are sweet, bland, and mild natured. We can apply a modified version of Harmonize the Six Decoction *(liù hé tāng)* from the Ming-dynasty book, *Five Texts by (Hu) Shen Rou (Shèn-Rǒu wǔ shū)* to treat this pattern:

Pseudostellariae Radix *(tài zǐ shēn)* 10g
Glehniae Radix *(běi shā shēn)* 10g
Poria *(fú líng)*... 10g
Dioscoreae Rhizoma *(shān yào)* 10g
Lablab Semen album *(bái biǎn dòu)* 10g
Mume Fructus *(wū méi)* flesh 10g
Paeoniae Radix alba *(bái sháo)*................................... 10g
Dendrobii Herba *(shí hú)* 10g
Atractylodis macrocephalae Rhizoma *(bái zhú)*............ 6g
Glycyrrhizae Radix *(gān cǎo)*..................................... 6g

After several packets, when the symptoms have begun to improve, the patient can also begin to eat a daily porridge made up of 30g of Dioscoreae Rhizoma *(shān yào)* and

6g of untreated Gigeriae galli Endothelium corneum *(jī nèi jīn)*, ground into a powder. The powder should be divided into two servings and taken each morning and evening. Mix the powder, combine with water, cook into a thick porridge, sweetened with sugar to taste, and eat. The patient should take the porridge for two weeks or longer. This porridge treatment is a unique approach to fortifying the Spleen and aiding its function of transportation. It is taken from the practice of the 20th-century physician Zhang Xi-Chun and is reliably effective.

Additionally, there is another pattern of food aversion in children seen in the clinic. This is Lung deficiency affecting the Spleen, a five-phase example of the child stealing the mother's qi (Lung/metal stealing qi from Spleen/earth). Symptoms include food aversion, pale complexion, weight loss, a weary or exhausted affect, dry cough, sweating when lying down, and dry stools. If examined, the lungs will not show any pathological changes. It is beneficial to treat both the Spleen and Lung together so that the child and mother mutually engender each other and lead both to a harmonious state of health. My custom is to use a modification of Zhang Xi-Chun's *Decoction to Restore Life (zī shēng tāng)*:

Dioscoreae Rhizoma *(shān yào)*	15g
Paeoniae Radix alba *(bái sháo)*	10g
untreated Fossilia Ossis Mastodi *(shēng lóng gǔ)*	10g
untreated Ostreae Concha *(shēng mǔ lì)*	10g
Atractylodis macrocephalae Rhizoma *(bái zhú)*	6g
Scrophulariae Radix *(xuán shēn)*	6g
Lycii Cortex *(dì gǔ pí)*	6g
dry-fried Arctii Fructus *(chǎo niú bàng zǐ)*	3g
Glycyrrhizae Radix *(gān cǎo)*	3g

This formula supports Spleen qi, boosts Stomach yin, nourishes Lung fluids, and binds up floating fire. In most cases, after 2-4 packets of the formula the patient's dry cough and night sweats will cease and their appetite will gradually improve.

4.4 Pediatric diarrhea

Child with five months of diarrhea

What is covered up by modern treatments?

現代治療掩蓋了什麼?

■ CASE HISTORY

Patient: *Ms. Wu, a 7-month-old girl*

INTAKE EXAMINATION

For the first two months of her life the child had relatively normal bowel movements. Later, due to being fed inappropriate food, the child developed diarrhea. Initially the child's bowel movements were watery and contained undigested food. Consequently, she was given two doses of Patchouli/Agastache Powder to Rectify the Qi *(huò xiāng zhèng qì sǎn)*, which was ineffective. She then took Western medicines, received injections and an intravenous drip, but nothing helped. Again, the parents turned to Chinese herbal medicine. During the following five months, the girl was given Preserve Harmony Pill *(bǎo hé wán)*, Ginseng, Poria, and White Atractylodes Powder *(shēn líng bái zhú sǎn)*, Aconite Accessory Root Pill to Regulate the Middle *(fù zǐ lǐ zhōng wán)*, True Man's Decoction to Nourish the Organs *(zhēn rén yǎng zàng tāng)*, and Four-Miracle Pill *(sì shén wán)*. Additionally, she had an herbal powder applied to her umbilicus, but her diarrhea continued.

Nine days prior to coming in to our clinic the child's condition had worsened, and she was having diarrhea, non-stop, night and day. The child was admitted to the hospital and diagnosed with 'simple indigestion'. Despite being on a continuous IV drip, as well as given medicines to fight infection and astringent, antidiarrheal medications over a period of nine days, the child's condition did not improve.

The girl's parents were worried sick and in a desperate situation. When they heard that our clinic had repeatedly cured prolonged pediatric diarrhea quickly with herbal medicine, they immediately carried their child to our clinic.

INTAKE EXAMINATION

DATE: afternoon of February 8, 1990

The patient's complexion was dusky-pale and her spirit and vitality were subpar. Her crying was soft and feeble, her lips were pale and lacked moisture. She was having diarrhea 10-20 times per day, more in the morning than the afternoon. Her stools were loose, like that of a duck's, and did not smell particularly bad. Her appetite was acceptable and urination was slightly decreased. Her tongue was pale red with a white coating that lacked moisture. The veins on her fingers were pale purple.

DIFFERENTIATION OF PATTERNS AND DISCUSSION OF TREATMENT

PHYSICIAN A   I cannot stop thinking about the issue of the pathodynamic in this case. What is the primary pathodynamic behind the diarrhea here, Dr. Yu?

DR. YU   Depletion of Spleen qi and Spleen yin due to chronic diarrhea. This depletion eventually led to the damage of Spleen yang.

PHYSICIAN B   The fact that the child's chronic diarrhea led to damage of Spleen qi and yang is evidenced by various symptoms. For example, her dusky-pale complexion, feeble crying, pale lips, and loose, duck-like stools all point to this diagnosis. However, there were virtually no signs of yin damage. If the child's yin had truly been damaged due to chronic diarrhea, there would have to be signs and symptoms like scanty, yellow urination, a decline in the suppleness of the child's skin, irritability, thirst, and a scarlet red tongue with scant moisture.

DR. YU   The primary reason there were not more obvious signs of yin damage was that the child received infusions for a long time. Infusions are a common method of treatment used in modern medicine. They can be important in treating urgent and life-threatening conditions and help to increase physical strength, but there are times when their use can mask the underlying conditions.

It is primarily for just this reason that it is quite unusual nowadays, in clinic, to see many of the nutritive or blood level symptoms associated with warm-heat disease that physicians from the warm disease school have described. It seems that this situation has created a fog of confusion around differential diagnosis. Do any of you have the same impression? As for this case, except for the fact that her lips and tongue lacked moisture, the patient, as you mentioned, had virtually no typical signs of yin damage. Consequently, the proposed existence of yin damage pathology was primarily based on the patient's medical history and consideration of the treatments she had been given.

PHYSICIAN C   I have read numerous articles on the subject of Spleen yin deficiency, and all of them have said that those with Spleen yin deficiency have dry stools. How is it that this child, who supposedly has Spleen yin damage, has incessant diarrhea?

DR. YU   It's my opinion that run-of-the-mill Spleen yin deficiency cannot be equated with damage to Spleen yin due to chronic diarrhea. First, diarrhea is invariably associated with dampness. So even though there was damage to Spleen yin, the fact that the child had incessant diarrhea indicated that a damp pathogen was present. Furthermore, the more depleted that the Spleen yin became, the more the Spleen qi was damaged. As the classics have said in Chapter 8 of the *Divine Pivot (Líng shū)*, "When yin is deficient, there is no qi." Hence, as the Spleen's ability to transport, transform, and deliver declines, the patient's diarrhea will continue to worsen. Since it is also true that as diarrhea worsens the patient's Spleen qi becomes weaker, a vicious cycle develops.

Based on the patient's medical history, past treatments and current symptoms, we determined that her pattern was one of long-term diarrhea depleting both Spleen qi and yin, which progressed to damaging the Spleen yang. Such a condition is benefited by a combination of Seven-Ingredient Powder with White Atractylodes *(qī wèi bái zhú sǎn)*, Enrich Yin and Clear Dryness Decoction *(zī yīn qīng zào tang)*, Regulate the Middle Decoction *(lǐ zhōng tāng)*, and Agrimony and Platycodon Root Decoction *(xiān hè tāng)*.

TREATMENT AND OUTCOME

Codonopsis Radix *(dǎng shēn)*	10g
Atractylodis macrocephalae Rhizoma *(bái zhú)*	10g
Poria *(fú líng)*	12g
Puerariae Radix *(gé gēn)*	10g
Pogostemonis/Agastaches Herba *(huò xiāng)*	10g
Aucklandiae Radix *(mù xiāng)*	6g
Glycyrrhizae Radix *(gān cǎo)*	10g
Dioscoreae Rhizoma *(shān yào)*	60g
Talcum *(huá shí)*	30g
Paeoniae Radix alba *(bái sháo)*	30g
Zingiberis Rhizoma *(gān jiāng)*	6g
Platycodi Radix *(jié gěng)*	10g
Agrimoniae Herba *(xiān hè cǎo)*	30g

Instructions: Soak the herbs in cold water for ten minutes. Cook at a low boil for one hour, until 200ml remains, strain and add sugar to taste. Divide into five doses and give the child one dose every hour. Continue to take any Western medicines as prescribed.

SECOND VISIT: (midday, February 9) The patient's father came to the clinic and reported that, because the medicine wasn't too bitter, they didn't have any difficulty getting the child to take it. She had finished the decoction the night before. He went on to say that early this morning her first bowel movement was basically formed, but three times after that her stools were loose, though somewhat drier than previously.

When a formula is effective, it should not be changed. The patient was given one more packet of the formula.

THIRD VISIT: (afternoon, February 10) The child's diarrhea had stopped. She had one bowel movement that day and it was completely formed. With great happiness her mother said, "In the past five months she hasn't once had a normal bowel movement like the one today." In order to consolidate the treatment, the patient was prescribed Fortify the Spleen syrup tablets *(jiàn pǐ gāo piàn)*. The formula is made by our hospital and essentially consists of Ginseng, Poria, and White Atractylodes Powder *(shēn líng bái zhú sǎn)* with sugar and 0.5g of raw herb in each tablet. The parents were told to give the girl two tablets, three times per day. They were to be chewed or finely ground up and taken with warm, boiled water. Six months later the family was contacted to see how the girl was doing. Her family said she had not had any recurrence of diarrhea since being released from the hospital and had gradually become more robust.

Disease	Primary symptoms	Differential diagnosis	Treatment method	Formula
Diarrhea	Immoderate diarrhea day and night	Long-term diarrhea depleting both Spleen qi and yin, progressing to damaging the Spleen yang	Enrich the yin, clear dryness while augmenting the qi and aiding the yin	Seven-Ingredient Powder with White Atractylodes *(qī wèi bái zhú sǎn)*, Enrich Yin and Clear Dryness Decoction *(zī yīn qīng zào tang)*, Regulate the Middle Decoction *(lǐ zhōng tāng)*, Agrimony and Platycodon Root Decoction *(xiān hè tāng)*

REFLECTIONS AND CLARIFICATIONS

PHYSICIAN A   This child had had diarrhea for five months, and besides taking Western medicines, had repeatedly taken Chinese medicines to disperse cold, reduce and guide out, strengthen the Spleen, warm the yang, and arrest and bind up. However, the diarrhea continued unabated. Given my limited experience, it seems to me a bit fortuitous that after giving her such a commonplace formula as a modified Seven-Ingredient Powder with White Atractylodes *(qī wèi bái zhú sǎn)*, suddenly, after just one bag, results were marked, and after two bags her symptoms had basically resolved.

DR. YU   Don't understand this case in terms of "a modified Seven-Ingredient Powder with White Atractylodes *(qī wèi bái zhú sǎn)*." What I prescribed was a complex prescription made up of four formulas: Seven-Ingredient Powder with White Atractylodes *(qī wèi bái zhú sǎn)*, Enrich Yin and Clear Dryness Decoction *(zī yīn qīng zào tang)*, Regulate the Middle Decoction *(lǐ zhōng tāng)*, and Agrimony and Platycodon Root Decoction *(xiān hè tāng)*. It is worth noting that the core of this compound formula is Enrich Yin and Clear Dryness Decoction *(zī yīn qīng zào tang)*, not Seven-Ingredient Powder with White Atractylodes *(qī wèi bái zhú sǎn)*.

PHYSICIAN A Saying "a modified Seven-Ingredient Powder with White Atractylodes *(qī wèi bái zhú sǎn)*" and saying "Seven-Ingredient Powder with White Atractylodes *(qī wèi bái zhú sǎn)* combined with three other formulas" is basically saying the same thing.

DR. YU In what way are those two things the same? The former refers to Seven-Ingredient Powder with White Atractylodes *(qī wèi bái zhú sǎn)* with the addition of a few other ingredients. The latter does not mean that at all. Most people understand that single herbs are usually added to address a specific symptom, whereas formulas are created to address a pathodynamic.

PHYSICIAN B As I understand your perspective Dr. Yu, the pathodynamic in this particular case is actually comprised of a complex of different pathodynamics, and thus requires a compound formula to address it in its entirety. The formula you prescribed contained four different formulas. Of those, Regulate the Middle Decoction *(lǐ zhōng tāng)* is the only one we are really familiar with. We don't know much about Seven-Ingredient Powder with White Atractylodes *(qī wèi bái zhú sǎn)*, and Enrich Yin and Clear Dryness Decoction *(zī yīn qīng zào tang)* and Agrimony and Platycodon Root Decoction *(xiān hè tāng)* are formulas that are unknown to most of us. Would you mind explaining a little bit more about these formulas?

DR. YU Seven-Ingredient Powder with White Atractylodes *(qī wèi bái zhú sǎn)* is comprised of Four-Gentlemen Decoction *(sì jūn zǐ tāng)* with the addition of Pogostemonis/Agastaches Herba *(huò xiāng)*, Aucklandiae Radix *(mù xiāng)*, and Puerariae Radix *(gé gēn)*. It originates in the Song-dynasty book by Qian Yi, *Craft of Medicines and Patterns for Children [Xiǎo ér yào zhèng zhēn jué]*. Qian Yi wrote:

> [This formula] treats long-term deficiency of the Spleen and Stomach, with persistent and frequent retching, vomiting, and diarrhea that has dried up and exhausted the essence and fluids with [symptoms such as] irritability and thirst. … This formula is suitable for such cases regardless of whether [the pattern] is yin or yang, excess or deficient.

Since the formula contains Four-Gentlemen Decoction *(sì jūn zǐ tāng)* it tonifies Spleen qi, while Pogostemonis/Agastaches Herba *(huò xiāng)* and Aucklandiae Radix *(mù xiāng)* drain turbid yin and direct it downward. Puerariae Radix *(gé gēn)*, on the other hand, raises clear qi. Furthermore, Puerariae Radix *(gé gēn)* is also able to engender fluids, relieve thirst, resolve heat in the muscular layer, and arrest diarrhea. Consequently, when diarrhea damages Spleen qi and Spleen yin, if the damage to yin is not extreme, this formula, used alone, can be very effective.

In this case, the child's diarrhea had continued for five months, the damage to Spleen yin was already severe, and so the formula was combined with Enrich Yin and Clear Dryness Decoction *(zī yīn qīng zào tang)* to greatly tonify Spleen yin. Enrich Yin and Clear Dryness Decoction *(zī yīn qīng zào tang)* comes from the great physician of the early part of the last century, Zhang Xi-Chun. It is found in his book *Essays on Medicine Esteeming the Chinese and Respecting the Western (Yī xué zhōng zhōng cān xī lù)*. Regarding Agrimony and Platycodon Root Decoction *(xiān hè tāng)* …

PHYSICIAN C   Dr. Yu, allow me to interrupt for a moment. I would like to request that you please clarify the issue of the treatment for Spleen yin damage. I have with me here a copy of *Essays on Medicine Esteeming the Chinese and Respecting the Western (Yī xué zhōng zhōng cān xī lù)*. First of all, the chapter containing Enrich Yin and Clear Dryness Decoction *(zī yīn qīng zào tang)*, which consists of Dioscoreae Rhizoma *(shān yào)* 30g, Talcum *(huá shí)* 30g, Paeoniae Radix alba *(bái sháo)* 12g, and Glycyrrhizae Radix *(gān cǎo)* 9g, does not clearly state that it treats chronic diarrhea with a pattern of Spleen yin damage. Secondly, TCM textbooks contain no discussion of long-term diarrhea damaging Spleen yin. What they say is that diarrhea "damages yin," and the recommended formula is Coptis and Mume Decoction *(lián méi tāng)*.

DR. YU   Textbooks cannot be expected to be written with all-encompassing detail. Nor can it be expected that a body will manifest an illness exactly like the patterns described in the textbooks. As for Zhang Xi-Chun never clearly stating that Enrich Yin and Clear Dryness Decoction *(zī yīn qīng zào tang)* can be used to treat damage to Spleen yin resulting from chronic diarrhea, this is true. However, a careful reading of his case studies using this formula, and his discussion of them, will certainly inspire some new perspectives.

For example, he says:

> A four-year-old child came down with warm disease. The pathogen was still in the exterior, but the doctor did not understand to clear heat and resolve the exterior and hastily gave the child a cold and bitter formula. After taking the formula the child had persistent diarrhea for four or five days. The upper burner was dry and hot, the child kept his eyes closed, he was wheezing, and his spirit was clouded. There was some delay before I could come and give a diagnosis and treatment, but although the disease was severe, the boy's pulse still had a root, so I knew that he could recover. I used Enrich Yin and Clear Dryness Decoction *(zī yīn qīng zào tang)* in its original form and advised that the formula be decocted down to an amount that would fill a large tea cup. Because he was so young, I recommended that the child drink the warm decoction slowly [throughout the day]. After finishing one bag the boy had recovered.

Dr. Zhang intentionally pointed out later in his discussion that this formula treated a pattern of "long-term diarrhea that exhausted yin." He went on to say:

> [If one only] clears the dry-heat then the diarrhea will intensify. [If one only] tonifies to treat diarrhea then the dry-heat will intensify. This formula contains Dioscoreae Rhizoma *(shān yào)* not only to stop diarrhea, but also to nourish yin and reduce heat. Talcum *(huá shí)* on the other hand promotes water metabolism and stops diarrhea. These two medicinal substances reinforce each other. Assisting these medicinal substances is Paeoniae Radix *(sháo yào)*, which nourishes yin blood and promotes urination, and Glycyrrhizae Radix *(gān cǎo)*, which not only harmonizes and regulates yin and yang and the central palace, but is also an essential herb for clearing heat and stopping diarrhea. When used together [these two substances] create an unusually effective formula. I have used this formula

numerous times to treat people [and have achieved] excellent results. Even in
very grave cases it can be effective.

What this means is that when treating a pattern of Spleen yin damage, substances to
nourish Spleen yin should be combined with those that promote water metabolism and
leach out dampness. Clinical experience shows substances that nourish yin without
hindering the expulsion of dampness and those that resolve dampness without damaging yin can be used together, and that rather than being in opposition, actually work
together to achieve remarkable results.

PHYSICIAN C   Regarding the ability of Enrich Yin and Clear Dryness Decoction *(zī yīn
qīng zào tang)* to treat a pattern of damage of Spleen yin due to chronic diarrhea, are
the results repeatable?

DR. YU   Yes they are. Let me be clear in saying that my knowledge that Enrich Yin and
Clear Dryness Decoction *(zī yīn qīng zào tang)* can treat this pattern and symptoms was
gained through much trial and error. In the early 1970s I was working in mountainous
regions, treating the local people whose staple food consisted primarily of low-grade
grains (corn, sorghum, millet). Because of this, and the fact that children's Spleens and
Stomachs are relatively underdeveloped, it was quite common for them to develop diarrhea. Add to that their poor economic conditions and lack of doctors and medicine,
and you will understand that cases of severe yin damage due to diarrhea were far from
rare. In fact, the children of the area would often have the typical signs and symptoms
of such a condition.

Initially, I would often give textbook formulas and herbs and the results were far
from ideal. After careful observation and reflection, I finally came to the realization that,
due to the various inherent differences in children's constitutions, this chronic condition could manifest with an array of yin damage signs and symptoms. These included
damage to Liver yin, Spleen yin, or Kidney yin. Treatment would primarily focus on
three formulas: Zanthoxyli and Mume Decoction *(jiāo méi tang)* for Liver yin damage,
Enrich Yin and Clear Dryness Decoction *(zī yīn qīng zào tang)* for Spleen yin damage,
and Coptis and Mume Decoction *(lián méi tāng)* for Kidney yin damage. The results
were very good, particularly when using Enrich Yin and Clear Dryness Decoction *(zī
yīn qīng zào tang)*. When I adjusted the doses of the herbs as follows: Dioscoreae Rhizoma *(shān yào)* 30-60g, Paeoniae Radix alba *(bái sháo)* 30g, Talcum *(huá shí)* 30g,
Glycyrrhizae Radix *(gān cǎo)* 9-15g, the effects were even more rapid. I summarized
my experience in an article, "Pattern Differentiation and Treatment: Yin Damage due
to Long-Term Diarrhea in Children," published in volume 2 of the *Journal of New
Chinese Medicine* in 1974.

Later, after I was dispatched to a hospital in the city, I discovered that an isolated
pattern of yin damage from chronic diarrhea was uncommon. The reason being that
people in the city usually get prompt treatment when ill, and often rely on infusions
from early on as part of their treatment. In fact, based on my observations, the spirit
and complexions of some patients with chronic persistent diarrhea were not far from
normal. However, it wasn't easy to get good results with these patients when using many
of the formulas and herbs typically used to treat chronic diarrhea. After analyzing many

medical histories and treatments, we realized that most of the cases showed signs of injury to all the major aspects of the Spleen: qi, yin, and yang. Most often the signs of injury to Spleen qi and Spleen yang were more evident, while the damage to Spleen yin was hidden or latent in most cases. From the manifestations we were able to grasp the nature of the patient's conditions, and employed the combined methods of tonifying Spleen qi, warming Spleen yang, nourishing Spleen yin, and promoting water metabolism and resolving dampness. The results were swift and effective.

PHYSICIAN C   Dr. Yu, you were talking about Agrimony and Platycodon Root Decoction *(xiān hè tāng)* when I interrupted you. Could you please continue that discussion?

DR. YU   Agrimony and Platycodon Root Decoction *(xiān hè tāng)* consists of two herbs, Agrimoniae Herba *(xiān hè cǎo)* and Platycodi Radix *(jié gěng)*. This formula comes from the Chinese medicine master of the second-half of the 20th century, Zhu Liang-Chun, and is based on his clinical experience treating chronic diarrhea. I simply incorporated it into my compound formula. I will also mention that these two herbs added to a formula for chronic persistent cough will greatly improve the results. Try it and see.

4.5.1 Pediatric coughing and wheezing

CASE 1: Childhood nighttime cough

Employ detailed questioning to rigorously pursue an understanding of the history of the patient's disease and treatment

窮追窮追細問病史與治療史

■ **CASE HISTORY**

Patient: *4-year-old boy*

This boy had been suffering from a nighttime cough for the past two months. Initially, he had caught a chill and then developed a cough that went on day and night. The boy was given Western drugs and an intravenous drip for seven days. After this, he no longer coughed during the day, but continued to cough at night.

Modifications of Inula Powder *(jīn fèi cǎo sǎn)* and Stop Coughing Powder *(zhǐ sòu sǎn)* were given for ten days along with the patent medicines Acute Bronchitis Syrup *(jí zhī táng jiāng)*[4] and Snake Bile and Aged Tangerine Peel Oral Liquid *(shé dǎn chén pí yè)* but the cough persisted. The patient had been given a chest x-ray and selected laboratory tests, but they revealed no signs of pathology.

....
4. This consists of Houttuyniae Herba *(yú xīng cǎo)*, *Fagopyrum dibotrys (jīn qiáo mài)*, Ilex purpurea *(sì jì qīng)*, Ephedrae Herba *(má huáng)*, Asteris Radix *(zǐ wǎn)*, Peucedani Radix *(qián hú)*, Aurantii Fructus *(zhǐ ké)*, and Glycyrrhizae Radix *(gān cǎo)*.

The child had seen numerous doctors. Some had posited that his pattern was one of Lung dryness and damage to the thin fluids, while others claimed that his condition was one of yang deficiency with exuberant fire. Still, none of the formulas he was given was effective. His condition continued unchanged for two months. His family, having heard that I had experience effectively treating difficult conditions, brought the child to see me.

Intake Examination
DATE: April 8, 1997

The boy was restless at night and had a frequent hacking cough that was most severe during the first half of the night. His appetite had markedly decreased, he had a dry mouth with a desire to drink, and dry stools. His tongue coating was thick, yellow, and greasy and he had a slippery and rapid pulse.

Differentiation of Patterns and Discussion of Treatment

PHYSICIAN A   The child's cough had dragged on for two months, and despite using both Western and Chinese medicines, his health had not improved. Tests showed no pathology in his lungs, yet the child's seemingly minor symptoms were very challenging to treat. It is no wonder that his parents were so frustrated. There is a folk saying that "famous doctors don't treat coughs or wheezing." It seems to me that if this is true, there are two reasons: first, since many people consider cough to be a minor ailment, resolving someone's cough doesn't seem like a very big achievement. Second, some coughs and wheezing are indeed difficult to treat and if the doctor fails to cure the patient, his or her family may be unforgiving and speak ill of the doctor's abilities.

DR. YU   I think we should carefully analyze the phrase "difficult to treat." Does it mean that coughing is truly difficult to treat, or is that only the case when it is not being treated correctly? Qing-dynasty physician Wu Ju-Tong emphasized that the key to attaining excellent results lies "wholly in accurately recognizing patterns." This case is an example of a cough that does not belong to the common categories seen in textbooks. Thus, based on my long experience in the clinic, I thought it might be the type of cough that is due to food accumulation.

It's actually quite easy to recognize a food-accumulation cough: a child contracts an external pathogen and develops a cough, has repeated treatments involving both Western and Chinese medicines, and even though the external pathogen resolves, the cough persists. The cough often lingers for a month or more and is accompanied by a distinctive symptom, such as during the daytime, the child's cough is less frequent or almost nonexistent, while it worsens at night. In addition, the child with this type of cough will experience fitful sleep and a mild feverishness. The child will often kick off their blankets or prefer sleeping with their arms and legs outside the blankets. Seeing such signs and symptoms, the practitioner should seriously consider whether the child has a case of food-accumulation cough and avoid continued use of customary formulas for stopping cough and transforming phlegm.

To ensure an accurate diagnosis, it is important to talk to the child's parents and gather detailed information about the child's diet and stools. Lastly, it is imperative to carefully check the appearance of the child's tongue. If the child's appetite is poor and the child has foul-smelling stools or constipation, and a reddish tongue with a yellow, greasy coating, more often than not this points to long-term food accumulation and stagnation, which has led to Stomach qi that is unable to properly descend and instead counterflows upward, assaulting the Lung and causing coughing.

PHYSICIAN B   After hearing Dr. Yu shed light on each aspect of this condition, it seems that identifying food-accumulation cough is an easy task. Yet when the patient is in front of you in the clinic it feels like a conundrum. It brings to mind the saying, "To be thoroughly familiar with Wang Shu-He[5] is not as good as having an abundance of clinical experience." This case is a good example. This young boy had a nocturnal cough that lingered for two months and didn't respond to either Western medications or Chinese herbs; his condition seemed to be untreatable. Yet for you, Dr. Yu, it was not a difficult case. You definitely diagnosed the child as having cough due to food accumulation and wrote a formula that brought quick results. Given that you are so familiar with this type of pediatric cough, you must have accumulated a wealth of experience in recognizing patterns; this knowledge is something worth passing on.

DR. YU   There are two important points to remember when seeing this type of patient in the clinic. First, a child who has a cough due to food accumulation won't necessarily have any obvious history that would predict food accumulation, such as a history of binging or overeating. They also may not have many, or any, symptoms of food accumulation, such as belching, acid reflux, or sensations of fullness and bloating in the chest or abdomen. If you don't ask detailed questions of the parents, you may overlook other relevant information. Second, many children with nighttime coughs will also present with heat in the palms and soles or have mild feverishness or low-grade fever during the night, which will lead many to wonder if the cough is due to yin deficiency. In his preface to the *Discussion of Cold Damage (Shāng hán lùn)*, Zhang Zhong-Jing made a remark that was critical of the physicians in his day, "[they are] with the patients for only a moment before they have decided on a formula." Quickly assuming these symptoms indicate yin deficiency and hastily prescribing medicinal substances to enrich yin and moisten the Lungs is being inattentive and perfunctory. The further along that path you venture, the worse the child's condition will become.

So, how do we differentiate between this type of cough and that of yin deficiency? First, in addition to meticulously asking about disease history and treatment history, the key is in the appearance of the tongue. Those with yin-deficiency cough have a tender, red tongue with no coating or only a scanty coating, and most definitely don't have a greasy coating. Contrariwise, those with cough due to food accumulation will have a yellow, greasy coating, which may be thick or thin. This is an indication of the turbidity and heat that rebels upward because of internal brewing of accumulated food.

PHYSICIAN B   If the situation is as you say, then it seems difficult to effectively treat food-accumulation cough with herbs alone.

....

5. Wang Shu-He is the third-century author of the *Pulse Classic (Mài jīng)* and was also an early editor of the works of Zhang Zhong-Jing.

DR. YU   Very true! When treating this condition, I don't rely solely on herbal medicine, but instead adhere to the principle laid out by Zhang Zhong-Jing. In line 398 of the *Discussion of Cold Damage (Shāng hán lùn)*, when referring to certain patients with weak Spleen and Stomach qi, he stated, "Reducing food [intake will] bring about a cure." What this means regarding food-accumulation cough is that the child's evening meal should be simplified as much as possible. Avoid high-protein and high-fat foods and other difficult-to-digest foodstuffs. A meal primarily consisting of vegetables is best. Avoiding snacks is also recommended. When combined with this 'dietary therapy', it is often possible that an herbal formula can achieve the traditional goal of "feeling a difference after one bag of herbs, resolution after two." Some parents, after their children were cured of these coughs, have looked me in the eye and said with great relief, "If we had known there could be results like this, we wouldn't have had to suffer through so many worthless medicines!"

TREATMENT AND OUTCOME

FIRST VISIT: The child had clear signs of cough due to food accumulation. The most appropriate treatment method would be to reduce the accumulated food, transform phlegm, clear heat, harmonize the Stomach and lead pathogens out of the body. We gave the child two packets of a modified version of a formula I created called Formula for Childhood Cough from Food Accumulation *(xiǎo ér shí jī ké sou fāng)*:

Bupleuri Radix *(chái hú)* 10g
Scutellariae Radix *(huáng qín)* 10g
standard Pinelliae Rhizoma praeparatum *(fǎ bàn xià)* 10g
Poria *(fú líng)* 15g
Aurantii Fructus *(zhǐ ké)* 10g
Atractylodis macrocephalae Rhizoma *(bái zhú)* 6g
Scorched Four Immortals:[6]
  – scorched Crataegi Fructus *(jiāo shān zhā)* 12g
  – scorched Hordei Fructus germinatus *(jiāo mài yá)* 12g
  – scorched Massa medicata fermentata *(jiāo shén qū)* 12g
  – scorched Gigeriae galli Endothelium corneum *(jiāo jī nèi jīn)* 12g
Forsythiae Fructus *(lián qiào)* 15g
wine-treated Rhei Radix et Rhizoma *(jiǔ zhì dà huáng)* ... [added near end] 3g

Instructions: Cook down to a concentrated form[7] and take frequently throughout the day. If the child is no longer constipated after taking the first packet, remove Rhei Radix et Rhizoma *(dà huáng)* from the second packet.

....

6. *Translators' note:* There are different formulations of this combination; the one noted here is the one used by Dr. Yu. If scorched Gigeriae galli Endothelium corneum *(jiāo jī nèi jīn)* is not available, scorched Setariae (Oryzae) Fructus germinatus *(jiāo gǔ yá)* can be used as a substitute.

7. *Translators' note:* This refers to a common way that decoctions are prepared for small children. The decoction is cooked normally and then the herbs are removed and the remaining liquid is cooked down to about one-half of its original volume. The child then takes a small amount of this concentrated liquid frequently, or alternatively 1-2 teaspoons every 2-3 hours.

SECOND VISIT:

Result: Twice that night, the child expelled foul-smelling stools. Following this, his cough was greatly diminished. After the second packet was finished, with Rhei Radix et Rhizoma *(dà huáng)* removed, the patient's yellow and greasy tongue coating was reduced by almost half. The child no longer wanted to drink as much and he became hungry and asked for food. During the middle of the night he only coughed a few times.

From this point on we switched to giving the child a modified Harmonize the Six Decoction *(liù hé tāng)*, a formula from *Five Texts from [Hu] Shen-Rou (Shèn-Róu wǔ shū)*. We prescribed four packets of the following:

Pseudostellariae Radix *(tài zǐ shēn)* 10g
Atractylodis macrocephalae Rhizoma *(bái zhú)* 6g
Poria *(fú líng)* 12g
Glycyrrhizae Radix *(gān cǎo)* 3g
Dioscoreae Rhizoma *(shān yào)* 12g
Lablab Semen album *(bái biǎn dòu)* 2g
Fritillariae thunbergii Bulbus *(zhè bèi mǔ)* 10g
Platycodi Radix *(jié gěng)* 6g
Armeniacae Semen *(xìng rén)* 10g
Eriobotryae Folium *(pí pá yè)* 15g

Result: The child's cough resolved and he slept peacefully through the night.

Disease	Primary symptoms	Differential diagnosis	Treatment method	Formula
Food-accumulation cough	Coughing during the night, thick, greasy, yellow tongue coating	Accumulation and stagnation of food and drink, leading to loss of proper downward movement of Stomach qi, which in turn rebels upward to assault the Lung	Disperse food accumulation and transform phlegm, clear heat and harmonize the Stomach, lead pathogens out of the body	Formula for Childhood Cough from Food Accumulation *(xiǎo ér shí jī ké sou fāng)*

REFLECTIONS AND CLARIFICATIONS

PHYSICIAN B   Dr. Yu, it looks like your Formula for Childhood Cough from Food Accumulation *(xiǎo ér shí jī ké sou fāng)* is actually a combination of Minor Bupleurum Decoction *(xiǎo chái hú tāng)* from *Discussion of Cold Damage (Shāng hán lùn)* plus Preserve Harmony Pill *(bǎo hé wán)* from the *Essential Teachings from [Zhu] Dan-Xi (Dān xī xīn fǎ)*. Is that correct?

DR. YU   It would be more accurate to call this formula a modification of a combination of Minor Bupleurum Decoction *(xiǎo chái hú tāng)* and Great Tranquility Pill *(dà ān wán)*, which is Preserve Harmony Pill *(bǎo hé wán)* plus Atractylodis macrocephalae Rhizoma *(bái zhú)*. Minor Bupleurum Decoction *(xiǎo chái hú tāng)* activates the pivot dynamic, thus raising the clear upward and directing the turbid downward. Great Tranquility Pill *(dà ān wán)* reduces accumulated food, guides it out of the body, improves the Spleen's transporting function and harmonizes the Stomach. The formula consists of:

Bupleuri Radix *(chái hú)* 10g

Scutellariae Radix *(huáng qín)* 6-10g

standard Pinelliae Rhizoma praeparatum *(fǎ bàn xià)* 10g

Poria *(fú líng)* 15g

Citri reticulatae Pericarpium *(chén pí)* 10g

Atractylodis macrocephalae Rhizoma *(bái zhú)* 10g

Scorched Four Immortals:

– scorched Crataegi Fructus *(jiāo shān zhā)* 12g

– scorched Hordei Fructus germinatus *(jiāo mài yá)* 12g

– scorched Massa medicata fermentata *(jiāo shén qū)* 12g

– scorched Gigeriae galli Endothelium corneum *(jiāo jī nèi jīn)* 12g

Forsythiae Fructus *(lián qiào)* 10-15g

The primary modifications are as follows:

- For extreme hacking cough, add 3g of honey-fried Ephedrae Herba *(má huáng)*, 6g of Belamcandae Rhizoma *(shè gān)*, and 10g of Stemonae Radix *(bǎi bù)* to dispel wind and benefit the throat. If this is ineffective it may be because the food-accumulation pattern is accompanied by exuberance of the Liver. In that case, instead of the previous additions, add 10g each of Cicadae Periostracum *(chán tuì)*, Bombyx batryticatus *(bái jiāng cán)*, and Pheretima *(dì lóng)* in order to pacify the Liver and resolve spasms.

- For patients whose stools tend to be dry, add 12g of Trichosanthis Semen *(guā lóu rén)* and 10g of Arctii Fructus *(niú bàng zǐ)* to clear heat and moisten the Intestines. If the constipation presents with clumped dried stool, add 3-5g of wine-treated Rhei Radix et Rhizoma *(jiǔ zhì dà huáng)* to discharge heat and unblock the bowels. Remove the Rhei Radix et Rhizoma *(dà huáng)* once the patient has had a bowel movement. When there is retching with the cough, add 6g of Zingiberis Rhizoma recens *(shēng jiāng)* and 10g of Bambusae Caulis in taeniam *(zhú rú)*, to direct rebellious qi downward and stop retching.

If the understanding of the pattern is accurate and the cough dramatically improves after taking 2-3 packets of the formula, yet a slight 'tail' of the cough remains, change to the experiential formula Eleven Herbs to Arrest Cough *(zhǐ ké shí yī wèi)*, which is 6g of each of the following:

Angelicae sinensis Radix *(dāng guī)*

wine-fried Chuanxiong Rhizoma *(jiǔ chǎo chuān xiōng)*

standard Pinelliae Rhizoma praeparatum *(fǎ bàn xià)*

Poria *(fú líng)*

Citri reticulatae Pericarpium *(chén pí)*

Glycyrrhizae Radix *(gān cǎo)*

Mori Cortex *(sāng bái pí)*

Citri reticulatae viride Pericarpium *(qīng pí)*

Schisandrae Fructus *(wǔ wèi zǐ)*

Armeniacae Semen *(xìng rén)*

Fritillariae thunbergii Bulbus *(zhè bèi mǔ)*

Two or three packets of these herbs should clear away this tail-end cough.

As I have said before,[8] even though the ingredients in this experiential formula are quite ordinary, in combination they become extraordinary. It's difficult to overstate their efficacy.

In cases where the patient's cough has resolved, but there are signs of insufficient qi and yin of the Spleen and Stomach, continue treatment with a suitably amended version of Harmonize the Six Decoction *(liù hé tāng)*[9] from the Song-dynasty work, *Five Texts from [Hu] Shen-Rou (Shèn-Róu wǔ shū)*. This will consolidate the treatment by enriching the Spleen and nourishing the Stomach.

PHYSICIAN A   Why do children with cough due to food accumulation mostly cough at night or experience coughing that is worse at night?

DR. YU   Daytime is yang, nighttime is yin, and yin governs stillness. This means that the functioning of the organs and bowels decreases during the night. Chinese medical theory suggests that children's organs are fragile [not fully developed], and the nocturnal functioning of the Spleen and Stomach is weaker than it is in adults. Food and drink aren't digested as easily and thus dampness accumulates and phlegm is produced. These rise and are stored in the Lung, causing pent-up Lung qi.

Chapter 38 of the *Basic Questions (Sù wèn)* states that overall, the pathodynamic of cough is one of pathological substances of phlegm and thin mucus, or water and dampness, "accumulating in the Stomach and lodging in the Lung." It would be entirely appropriate to use this statement to explain pediatric cough due to food accumulation.

PHYSICIAN B   In this case the child's cough was worse during the first half of the night. Is this usually the case?

DR. YU   Yes it is. In most cases the child's cough is worse during the first half of the night, sometime shortly after dinner, particularly when the child has eaten something that is difficult to digest. This would put some strain on the Spleen and Stomach, don't you think? Occasionally, the child's cough will worsen early in the morning. Tang Zong-Hai, a late 19th-century physician from Sichuan, wrote in his book, *Discussion of Blood Patterns (Xuè zhèng lùn)*, "The fire from food accumulation enters the Lung channel during the *yín* 寅 time." *Yín* is one of the 12 earthly branches and *yín* time refers to the time between 3 and 5 a.m. In traditional phase energetics, 3 to 5 a.m. is the time governed by the hand *tài yīn* Lung channel.

PHYSICIAN B   If that is the time period governed by the Lung channel, then Lung qi should be strong at that time. Isn't it logical to assume that there shouldn't be coughing at that time?

....

8. *A Walk Along the River*, vol. 1, p. 18.

9. This consists of Pseudostellariae Radix *(tài zǐ shēn)*, Atractylodis macrocephalae Rhizoma *(bái zhú)*, Poria *(fú líng)*, Glycyrrhizae Radix *(gān cǎo)*, Dioscoreae Rhizoma *(shān yào)*, and Lablab Semen album *(bái biǎn dòu)*.

DR. YU   Fire from food accumulation enters the Lung channel during the *yīn* time, but if the Lungs are strong, they will reject pathogens. It is through intense coughing that the Lungs expel the phlegm-fire pathogens that are attacking them. This is a self-protective mechanism of the body.

PHYSICIAN A   Regarding food-accumulation cough, there is no clear record of this illness in any ancient medical texts, nor any examples of this pattern in any modern college Chinese medicine textbook. In recent years, there has been the occasional article written on the subject, but these articles center on the theory of Spleen and Lung deficiency, while treatment methods stress simultaneous tonification of the Spleen and Lung, or nurturing of earth to generate metal. This is completely different than the pattern you have set forth for us here. How can we reconcile this?

DR. YU   I am also aware of these scattered clinical reports. Objectively speaking, there is no lack of discussion in the ancient literature about chronic cough in children due to Spleen and Lung deficiency, or due to earth failing to generate metal. Modern biomedicine considers this is a type of pediatric immunodeficiency where children readily catch colds and have repeated upper respiratory tract infections. This falls under the scope of a type of 'susceptibility syndrome' which has also been called refractory cough. There have been acceptable results gained from tonifying both the Spleen and Lung, or nurturing earth to generate metal, with formulas such as a modified combination of Six-Gentlemen Decoction *(liù jūn zǐ tāng)* plus Cinnamon Twig Decoction *(guì zhī tāng)* and Jade Windscreen Powder *(yù píng fēng sǎn)*.

Different people have different views. This may just be a variant pattern of food-accumulation cough. Nevertheless, the type of food-accumulation cough I described previously is very easy to differentiate. Most doctors of traditional Chinese medicine wouldn't misdiagnose and thus mistreat this type of cough.

PHYSICIAN A   Modern textbooks of traditional Chinese medicine already clearly classify cough due to concurrent Spleen and Lung deficiency, or earth not generating metal, as falling within the category of cough due to internal damage. I am unclear whether the food-accumulation cough that you are referring to is a type of external-contraction cough or an internal-damage cough.

DR. YU   Clinically speaking, it's very difficult to separate the two; or we can say that sometimes external contraction and internal damage can occur together. Over many years I have observed that if a child with a long-term intemperate diet has a cough that has damaged his or her Spleen and Stomach but doesn't contract an external pathogen, they will get better by themselves. However, when a child with a compromised Spleen and Stomach does contract an external pathogen, any problems will become entrenched and frequently linger.

In other situations, even though the external pathogen has temporarily been eliminated, the food accumulation still exists and the Stomach's ability to receive food and the Spleen's ability to transport essence are both diminished. As a result, food and drink cannot be properly transformed into refined essence, and time and time again, dampness gathers and generates phlegm. If the source of phlegm has not been cleared up, how can the storehouse of phlegm be clear and empty? The proper method for treating childhood cough due to food accumulation consists of strengthening the Spleen's ability to transport, harmonizing the Stomach and leading pathogens out of the body.

My own Formula for Childhood Cough from Food Accumulation (*xiǎo ér shí jī ké sou fāng*) contains Minor Bupleurum Decoction (*xiǎo chái hú tāng*) within it. This is the chief formula for treating *shào yáng* disease and was first mentioned in the chapter on *tài yáng* disease in the *Discussion of Cold Damage (Shāng hán lùn)*. The reason for its appearance in this chapter is that Minor Bupleurum Decoction (*xiǎo chái hú tāng*) can activate the *shào yáng* pivot. From the pivot of *shào yáng* reaching outward to the qi of *tài yáng*, the pathogenic qi is led out of the body. While I was exploring which formulas I could use to treat childhood food-accumulation cough I gave great weight to the unique ability of Minor Bupleurum Decoction (*xiǎo chái hú tāng*) to concurrently treat both external contraction and internal damage.

4.5.2 Pediatric coughing and wheezing

CASE 2: Child with coughing and wheezing for one month

The true mindset of one treading on thin ice

如履薄冰的真實心態

■ CASE HISTORY

Patient: *8-week-old boy*

The patient was born a month premature. When he was 20 days old, he developed pneumonia. After 14 days in the hospital the boy's health had improved enough that he was discharged. A few days later he once again began to cough and wheeze.

Before coming to my clinic, the boy had taken many packets of Ephedra, Apricot Kernel, Gypsum, and Licorice Decoction (*má xìng shí gān tāng*), which had helped his condition. However, his symptoms returned once he stopped taking the decoction, and although he did not have a fever, his condition worsened each day. During his course of treatment, the boy had been given numerous injections, as well as oral Western medicines, IV infusions and oxygen therapy, but nothing seemed to help. There were several times his condition became particularly grave.

He was given a biomedical diagnosis of asthmatic pneumonia and congenital heart disease (atrial septal defect). At this point the child's parents felt there was nothing that could be done except to seek help in the hospital's Chinese medicine department.

INTAKE EXAMINATION
DATE: June 2, 1986

The boy appeared listless. His complexion was dusky-pale, his lips were cyanotic, and he was emaciated. His breathing was labored, with coughing and wheezing and a gurgling sound from phlegm in his throat. He made sounds somewhere between moaning and crying and was dripping with cold sweat. During the night, his sleep was restless and periodically he would become agitated, have mild convulsions, and his extremities would become icy cold. The child was difficult to breastfeed and his stools were filled with partially digested milk. His tongue was pale with a white coating and the veins on his index fingers were pale red.

DIFFERENTIATION OF PATTERNS AND DISCUSSION OF TREATMENT

PHYSICIAN A   The child in this case has asthmatic pneumonia and presents with numerous signs and symptoms that indicate a very severe condition that involves a complex of pathodynamics. My concern is that if one were not extremely cautious in such a situation it could be easy to make mistakes with the treatment. How did you clearly grasp the pathodynamic here?

DR. YU   Using inductive reasoning this is clear at a glance. Let's look at the patient's symptoms according to pathodynamics.

1. A premature birth indicates congenital insufficiency. The child's cough and wheezing had continued for a month despite repeated attempts to treat him with Western medicines. He had a listless spirit, dusky-white complexion, cyanotic lips, dripping cold sweats, agitation, convulsions, cold limbs and pale-red veins on his index finger. These are all clear signs that the boy's condition is one of Heart yang deficiency.

2. The boy appeared emaciated and he resisted eating or breastfeeding; his stools contained undigested food. This clearly indicates that his Stomach is deficient and unable to take in food while the Spleen is deficient and unable to transport food essence.

3. The patient's coughing, wheezing, and dyspnea with distinct gurgling from phlegm in his airway reveals that the boy has phlegm counterflowing upward and attacking the Lung.

The first two groups of symptoms indicate deficient normal qi, while the third group of symptoms points to an overwhelming abundance of pathogenic qi.

PHYSICIAN B   Given that the overall pattern is deficient normal qi and overwhelming abundance of pathogenic qi, it would be logical to support normal qi and dispel the pathogen. How does one select a formula and specific herbs to address this situation?

DR. YU   First, to avoid making fundamental errors as you select herbs and formulas, it is important to clearly grasp the fundamental pathodynamics and treatment principles of the case. I cannot emphasize enough how important this is in the clinical setting. The specific treatment principle should be based on the specific pathodynamic. Only when the treatment principle is firmly established can one proceed with a finely developed approach.

The specific pathodynamics in this case are exhaustion of Heart yang, encumbered and exhausted Spleen and Stomach qi, and counterflow ascent of phlegm qi. The specific treatment principle is to warm and fortify Heart yang, assist the transportive functions of the Spleen, harmonize the Stomach, dispel phlegm, and direct counterflow qi downward.

Because the patient's Heart yang deficiency is acute and severe, starting with warming and fortifying Heart yang to save him from this critical condition should be the focus of treatment.

There are several factors affecting the increase in severity of the patient's illness. The child started out with a weak constitution, and for a long time his normal qi had been unsuccessfully battling pathogenic qi. This ongoing battle damaged both yin and yang. The child's Lung, which, having been fettered by wind and cold, lost its ability to disseminate qi and direct it downward. In addition to this, the boy's Heart yang was weak and the ability of his Spleen to transport was hampered. His normal qi weakened by the day, leaving him with this recalcitrant and critical condition.

TREATMENT AND OUTCOME

The *Discussion of Cold Damage (Shāng hán lùn)* states in line 18, "When a a patient who habitually wheezes has an attack, Cinnamon Twig Decoction *(guì zhī tāng)* plus Magnoliae officinalis Cortex *(hòu pò)* and Armeniacae Semen *(xìng rén)* is best." Hence, I gave the boy an augmented version of Cinnamon Twig Decoction plus Magnolia Bark and Apricot Kernel *(guì zhī jiā hòu pò xìng zǐ tāng)*, which transforms qi, adjusts yin and yang, directs qi downward, and halts wheezing:

Cinnamomi Ramulus *(guì zhī)*..3g
Paeoniae Radix alba *(bái sháo)*...6g
Glycyrrhizae Radix *(gān cǎo)*..3g
Jujubae Fructus *(dà zǎo)* 10g
Zingiberis Rhizoma recens *(shēng jiāng)*...............................2 slices
Magnoliae officinalis Cortex *(hòu pò)*.................................10g
Armeniacae Semen *(xìng rén)* 6g
Perillae Fructus *(zǐ sū zǐ)*...10g
Sinapis Semen *(bái jiè zǐ)*...5g
dry-fried Raphani Semen *(lái fú zǐ)*......................................6g
Lepidii/ Descurainiae Semen *(tíng lì zǐ)* 6g
Astragali Radix *(huáng qí)*...15g
Atractylodis macrocephalae Rhizoma *(bái zhú)*......................6g
Poria *(fú líng)*...6g

The strained decoction was given to the patient using an infant medicine dropper. That night, after finishing one packet of the formula, the boy sweat profusely and his coughing, wheezing, dyspnea, and cold sweats were all greatly reduced. He was then able to sleep peacefully. After finishing his second packet of herbs, the boy ate easily, his bowel movements normalized, and his complexion and lips became a normal pink. Only his cough remained. He was given three packets of the same formula, but this time I removed the Raphani Semen *(lái fú zǐ)* and added:

Inulae Flos *(xuán fù huā)* [separately decocted in a bag] 3g
Platycodi Radix *(jié gěng)* 6g
standard Pinelliae Rhizoma preparatum *(fǎ bàn xià)*...............6g

After finishing this prescription the symptoms had completely resolved. His spirit was lively, he had a rosy complexion, his appetite increased, his sleep was excellent, and urination and bowel movements were normal. The only symptoms that remained were a slight cough and a profuse discharge from his left eye. I prescribed two packets of Inula Powder *(jīn fèi cǎo sǎn)* plus Chrysanthemi Flos *(jú huā)*, Forsythiae Fructus *(lián qiáo)* and Mori Folium *(sāng yè)*. After this the boy's respiratory problems were no longer an issue.[10]

Note: After he recovered, the boy's family took him to the West China Center of Medical Sciences at Sichuan University to get a physical exam. Doctors there said there was no evidence to show that the boy had any congenital heart disease. At the time of this writing the boy was five years old and in good health.

Disease	Primary symptoms	Differential diagnosis	Treatment principle	Formulas
Cough and wheezing	Cough with wheezing, profuse cold sweats, refusal to breastfeed	Heart yang deficiency, encumbered and exhausted Spleen and Stomach, counterflow ascent of phlegm-qi attacking the Lung	Warm and fortify Heart yang, promote the Spleen's ability to transport and transform, harmonize the Stomach, dispel phlegm and redirect counterflow qi downward	A combination of Cinnamon Twig Decoction plus Magnolia Bark and Apricot Kernel *(guì zhī jiā hòu pò xìng zǐ tāng)*, Poria, Cinnamon Twig, Atractylodes, and Licorice Decoction *(líng guì zhú gān tāng)*, Three-Seed Decoction to Nourish One's Parents *(sān zǐ yǎng qīn tāng)*, and Descurainia and Jujube Decoction to Drain the Lung *(tíng lì dà zǎo xiè fèi tāng)*

REFLECTIONS AND CLARIFICATIONS

PHYSICIAN A   This child's case was very severe. He was only 20 days old when he became sick and had been repeatedly treated with Western medicines. In addition to all that, he had already been sick for one month before he came to see you. Were you absolutely confident of your diagnosis?

DR. YU   Honestly speaking, I was actually not that confident and certainly would not use the word "absolutely." Even though I prescribed two packets of the formula I was quite nervous about the situation. I specifically told the boy's parents that they were to bring him back to see me after he finished one packet of the formula. The following day my students and I waited on pins and needles for his return. It wasn't until about ten in the morning, when the family suddenly appeared and happily reported that he was feeling better, that we knew the medicine had hit its target and we all breathed a sigh of relief. It was only then that I told them to give their son the second packet. Things went smoothly after that.

PHYSICIAN C   Since warming and fortifying Heart yang was the emphasis of the treatment, why did you use a modification of Cinnamon Twig Decoction plus Magnolia Bark and

....

10. This case was included in Jiang Er-Xun and Long Zhi-Ping, eds. *Applied Research of Cinnamon Twig Decoction Formula Family Patterns* (桂枝湯類方證應用研究 *guì zhī tang lèi fang zhèng yìng yòng yán jiū*). Chengdu: Sichuan Science and Technology Press (1989), 87-88.

Apricot Kernel *(guì zhī jiā hòu pò xìng zǐ tāng)*? The formula only adjusts the nutritive and protective qi, dispels phlegm, and directs qi downward. I have never heard it said that the formula can warm and fortify Heart yang.

DR. YU   My perspective has been influenced and inspired by my teacher, Jiang Er-Xun. Dr. Jiang devoted much of his time in recent years to delving deeply into the fundamental formula patterns of the *Discussion of Cold Damage (Shāng hán lùn)*. He has written articles expressing his unique perspective about the theory underlying Cinnamon Twig Decoction *(guì zhī tāng)* formula-pattern and about clinical research of the formula. Dr. Jiang summarized his beliefs about the ancient masters' use of Cinnamon Twig Decoction *(guì zhī tāng)* by saying, "When used during an external pattern, it resolves the muscle layer and harmonizes the nutritive and protective qi. When used with an internal pattern, it transforms qi and adjusts yin and yang." This is not empty talk.

Dr. Jiang looked at Cinnamon Twig Decoction *(guì zhī tāng)* as an amalgamation of Cinnamon Twig and Licorice Decoction *(guì zhī gān cǎo tāng)* and Peony and Licorice Decoction *(sháo yào gān cǎo tāng)*. Cinnamon Twig and Licorice Decoction *(guì zhī gān cǎo tāng)* combines acrid and sweet flavors, which together transform yang, whereas Peony and Licorice Decoction *(sháo yào gān cǎo tāng)* combines sour and sweet flavors, which in tandem transform yin. Together, these two formulas adjust and harmonize yin and yang for both external and internal patterns. Cinnamon Twig Decoction *(guì zhī tāng)* is the formula best able to bring about an integrated adjustment.

Line 18 of the *Discussion of Cold Damage (Shāng hán lùn)* [translated above] refers to those people who have an inherent deficiency and disharmony of yin and yang (which includes protective and nutritive qi, as well as qi and blood). If a person of this constitutional type, with latent asthma, contracts an external pathogen that induces an attack of wheezing, the most suitable formula is Cinnamon Twig Decoction plus Magnolia Bark and Apricot Kernel *(guì zhī jiā hòu pò xìng zǐ tāng)*. This formula will dispel phlegm and direct qi downward. Zhang Zhong-Jing's observation that this variation of the formula "is best" means that the formula's effects have withstood the test of time in the clinic.

On reflection, at the time I was merely following the thought process of Dr. Jiang in prescribing this formula. However, the formula only conformed to the underlying pathodynamic—deficient normal qi and exuberant pathogenic qi—without completely addressing the specific pathodynamic of the patient's condition. Consequently, I went to Dr. Jiang to ask for his help with the case. I showed Dr. Jiang my formula, and after a moment of deep thought he added Atractylodis macrocephalae Rhizoma *(bái zhú)*, Poria *(fú líng)*, and Astragali Radix *(huáng qí)*, which made the formula a combination of Cinnamon Twig Decoction plus Magnolia Bark and Apricot Kernel *(guì zhī jiā hòu pò xìng zǐ tāng)* and Poria, Cinnamon Twig, Atractylodes, and Licorice Decoction *(líng guì zhú gān tāng)* plus Astragali Radix *(huáng qí)*. This combination creates a formula that effectively warms and fortifies Heart yang.

Later, after reviewing the diagnosis, Dr. Jiang added Perillae Fructus *(zǐ sū zǐ)*, Sinapis Semen *(bái jiè zǐ)*, Raphani Semen *(lái fú zǐ)*, and Lepidii/ Descurainiae Semen *(tíng lì zǐ)*, based on Three-Seed Decoction to Nourish One's Parents *(sān zǐ yǎng qīn tāng)* and Descurainia and Jujube Decoction to Drain the Lung *(tíng lì dà zǎo xiè fèi tāng)*. Such a combination not only improves the transportive functions of the Spleen and harmonizes the Stomach, but also increases the body's ability to expel phlegm and direct qi downward.

You can see then that, despite me saying the formula is a modification of Cinnamon Twig Decoction plus Magnolia Bark and Apricot Kernel *(guì zhī jiā hòu pò xìng zǐ tāng)*, within this one prescription there are actually three additional formulas: Poria, Cinnamon Twig, Atractylodes, and Licorice Decoction *(líng guì zhú gān tāng)*, Three-Seed Decoction to Nourish One's Parents *(sān zǐ yǎng qīn tāng)*, and Descurainia and Jujube Decoction to Drain the Lung *(tíng lì dà zǎo xiè fèi tāng)*. To reiterate, this combination warms and fortifies Heart yang, improves the Spleen's transportive functions, harmonizes the Stomach, dispels phlegm, and directs qi downward.

Physician B   The formula you prescribed was very effective and worth remembering for the future. Nevertheless, I can't help but wonder if the formula might be suitable for just this one case. According to the patient's history, he had previously shown improvement after having taken a few packets of Ephedra, Apricot Kernel, Gypsum, and Licorice Decoction *(má xìng shí gān tāng)*. However, after stopping the medication his symptoms returned. My question is, why didn't you continue along the same line as the previous doctor? After all, aren't coughing and wheezing, shortness of breath, and breaking a cold sweat precisely the symptoms associated with Ephedra, Apricot Kernel, Gypsum, and Licorice Decoction *(má xìng shí gān tāng)*?

DR. YU   Line 63 of the *Discussion of Cold Damage (Shāng hán lùn)* states that, "After inducing sweating one should not again utilize Cinnamon Twig Decoction *(guì zhī tāng)*. If there is sweating and wheezing without intense fever, Ephedra, Apricot Kernel, Licorice and Gypsum Decoction *(má huáng xìng rén gān cǎo shí gāo tang)* can be used." If we try to understand the pattern through the composition of the formula we come to see that the wheezing referred to in this passage is due to pathogenic qi obstructing the Lung. Thus, Ephedrae Herba *(má huáng)* is combined with Armeniacae Semen *(xìng rén)* to disseminate Lung qi and resolve the obstruction. The sweating in this pattern is due to constrained Lung heat. Ephedrae Herba *(má huáng)* and Gypsum fibrosum *(shí gāo)* are paired to disseminate Lung qi and drain heat. Ephedra, Apricot Kernel, Gypsum, and Licorice Decoction *(má xìng shí gān tāng)* uses acrid and cool medicinal substances to disseminate Lung qi, drain heat, clear the Lung and calm wheezing. It is a formula designed to treat wheezing and cough due to excess heat.

For the formula to be effective during the initial stages of the patient's illness, the symptoms of that pattern had to be present. However, after the patient stopped taking the herbs, not only did his symptoms return, but they worsened over time. Even though he was still coughing and wheezing, the boy's simple cold sweats had developed into copious, dripping cold sweats with a series of other signs indicating Heart yang deficiency. What this indicates is that his wheezing pattern had transformed from one of excess into one of deficiency. If, as you suggest, we continued with Ephedra, Apricot Kernel, Gypsum, and Licorice Decoction *(má xìng shí gān tāng)* because it was initially effective, then we would have committed the error of further depleting an already deficient condition.

There is currently a trend in China of "painting by numbers" with herbal medicine, that is, using a specific formula to address a specific biomedical diagnosis. Many physicians, for example, will immediately think of Ephedra, Apricot Kernel, Gypsum, and Licorice Decoction *(má xìng shí gān tāng)* the moment they face a patient who has pneumonia. Identifying a pattern based solely on the biomedical diagnosis, as well as the habit of using herbs and formulas perfunctorily while neglecting to carefully examine the details of the patient's case, goes against the fundamental principle of determining the treatment based on differential diagnosis.

4.6 Pediatric whooping cough

Child with whooping cough for one month

Breaking out from the confines of textbooks

冲出教科书的"樊籠"

■ CASE HISTORY

Patient: *5-year-old boy*

This young boy had developed a cough that appeared, in its initial stages, to be externally contracted. He had taken four packets of a modified Inula Powder *(jīn fèi cǎo sǎn)*, but it was ineffective. His cough gradually became worse until he developed a spasmodic, hacking cough so severe that his coughing fits of dozens of coughs in a row would bring tears to his eyes. Near the end of these coughing fits, he would invariably gasp once deeply for air, emitting a whooping sound. Then, with all his might, he would cough up some sticky sputum. When especially severe, he would also spit up food particles. These coughing fits would occur about ten times per day.

The child had been diagnosed with whooping cough by Western doctors and given a week's worth of Western medicine that had been ineffective.

The Chinese medicine diagnosis was paroxysmal cough (頓咳 *dùn ké*). He was first treated with four packets of a formula that combined Drain the White Powder *(xiè bái sǎn)* and Reed Decoction *(wěi jīng tāng)*. This was followed by three packets of a combination of Fritillaria and Trichosanthes Fruit Powder *(bèi mǔ guā lóu sǎn)* and Mori Cortex Decoction *(sāng bái pí tāng)*, taken along with a single chicken gallbladder consumed once per day. After taking this combination for a week, there was no clear amelioration of the persistent, spasmodic, hacking cough.

INTAKE EXAMINATION
DATE: January 20, 1985

The boy was brought to Dr. Yu by Physician B after Physician B failed to improve the patient's condition. In addition to the aforementioned symptoms, the young boy was listless, his eyes were puffy, and the inside of his eyelids were red. His tongue was red with a thin, yellow coating, and his pulse was fine and rapid.

DIFFERENTIATION OF PATTERN AND DISCUSSION OF TREATMENT

PHYSICIAN A   Paroxysmal cough is another name for whooping cough and is generally seen only in children. Because it is highly contagious, it has historically also been referred to as 'epidemic cough' (疫咳 *yì ké*).

In recent years China has seen a dramatic reduction in cases of whooping cough due to the widespread use of vaccines. However, cases of the illness still occur periodically in rural areas. Once a patient enters the paroxysmal phase characterized by a persistent and spasmodic cough, it becomes a thorny problem for both Chinese and Western medicine. In severe cases, patients may concurrently develop pneumonia, and in a worst-case scenario, seizures.

From a theoretical standpoint, one strives for an early diagnosis so that the child can be quarantined and timely treatment can begin. Clinically speaking, however, at the present time there are no medicines that can nip the illness in the bud. Patients, their families and doctors can only watch the illness gradually proceed into its paroxysmal phase when the characteristic spasmodic cough and whooping begins.

PHYSICIAN B   From my experience, I know it can be difficult to distinguish the early stages of whooping cough from a common externally-contracted cough, and often whooping cough ends up being treated as a typical externally-contracted cough. I myself have mistakenly treated a few cases of whooping cough as if it were a simple externally-contracted cough, and was thus unsuccessful. Gradually the patients would begin to cough more and more frequently until they developed the persistent and spasmodic coughing that is typical of the illness. They would also develop the 'whooping' sound that comes from long and deep inhalations after each bout of coughing. It wasn't until now that I understand that whooping cough is traditionally known in Chinese medicine as paroxysmal cough.

This boy was my patient and before I brought him to you, based on what was written in *The Collected Treatises of [Zhang] Jing Yue*, I prescribed a modification of Mori Cortex Decoction *(sāng bái pí tāng)*—Mori Cortex *(sāng bái pí)*, Pinelliae Rhizoma preparatum *(zhì bàn xià)*, Perillae Fructus *(zǐ sū zǐ)*, Armeniacae Semen *(xìng rén)*, Fritillariae Bulbus *(bèi mǔ)*, Scutellariae Radix *(huáng qín)*, Coptidis Rhizoma *(huáng lián)*, Gardeniae Fructus *(zhī zǐ)*—to drain the lungs and suppress the cough. The results were poor.

I also tried various other formulas, including a formula written by Song-dynasty physician Qian Yi called Drain the White Powder *(xiè bái sǎn)*, to drain and clear Lung heat; Ophiopogonis Decoction *(mài mén dōng tāng)*, from the Tang-dynasty work *Important Formulas Worth a Thousand Gold Pieces* (*Qiān jīn yào fāng*), to moisten dryness and direct rebellious qi downward; and Reed Decoction *(wěi jīng tāng)*, another formula from *Important Formulas Worth a Thousand Gold Pieces* (*Qiān jīn yào fāng*), to clear the Lung and dislodge phlegm. The efficacy of all these formulas was disappointing. As the saying goes, "Obtaining a thousand formulas is easy, but getting a single good result is difficult."

Treatment and Outcome

DR. YU   I considered the patient's pattern to be one of toxicity damaging the Liver and Kidneys, with Liver fire punishing the Lung. Treatment includes nourishing the Liver and restraining fire, enriching the Kidneys and resolving toxicity, moistening the Lung and dislodging phlegm. I prescribed a modification of Master Jian's Whooping Cough Formula (*Jiǎn shì dùn ké fāng*):

Paeoniae Radix alba *(bái sháo)* 20g
Glycyrrhizae Radix *(gān cǎo)* 10g
Schisandrae Fructus *(wǔ wèi zǐ)* 6g
Coptidis Rhizoma *(huáng lián)* 3g
Pheretima *(dì lóng)* 10g
Cicadae Periostracum *(chán tuì)* 10g
Scrophulariae Radix *(xuán shēn)* 15g
Ophiopogonis Radix *(mài mén dōng)* 15g
Glehniae Radix *(běi shā shēn)* 15g
Ostreae Concha *(mǔ lì)* 30g
Woodwardiae Rhizoma *(gǒu jǐ guàn zhòng)*[11] 15g
Bombyx batryticatus *(bái jiāng cán)* 10g
artificial Bambusae Concretio silicea *(rén gōng tiān zhú huáng)* 12g

The patient was given seven packets of herbs, one packet taken each day. In addition, I prescribed 25g each of Scolopendra *(wú gōng)* and Glycyrrhizae Radix *(gān cǎo)*. The two substances were to be combined and ground together. Two grams of the mixture were to be combined with honey and taken three times per day.

After taking four packets of herbs the boy's spasmodic, hacking cough had markedly improved, and after the sixth packet his cough had completely resolved. He did not take the last packet of herbs.

I prescribed Glehnia and Ophiopogonis Decoction *(shā shēn mài mén dōng tāng)* with Four-Gentlemen Decoction *(sì jūn zǐ tāng)* to complete his recovery.

Disease	Primary symptoms	Differential diagnosis	Treatment method	Formula
Paroxysmal cough (whooping cough)	Spasmodic, hacking cough with a long, deep intake of air and whooping	Toxicity damaging the Liver and Kidneys, with Liver fire punishing the Lung	Nourish the Liver and restrain fire; enrich the Kidneys and resolve toxicity; moisten the Lung and dislodge phlegm	Master Jian's Whooping Cough Formula (*Jiǎn shì dùn ké fāng*)

Reflections and Clarifications

PHYSICIAN A   Dr. Yu, your effective use of a modified Master Jian's Whooping Cough Formula (*Jiǎn shì dùn ké fāng*) to treat paroxysmal cough is indicative of your great depth

---

11. *Translators' note:* Woodwardiae Rhizoma (狗脊贯众 *gǒu jǐ guàn zhòng*) is a bitter and cold herb that is used to clear heat, resolve toxicity, kill parasites, stop bleeding, and expel wind-dampness. This has similar functions to the group of herbs known as *guàn zhòng* (Dryopteridis/Cyrtomii/etc. Rhizoma).

of knowledge. However, your description of the pathodynamic, "toxicity damaging the Liver and Kidneys with Liver fire punishing the Lung," sounds rather unusual. Particularly the five words "toxicity damaging the Liver and Kidneys." What is the basis for summarizing the pathodynamic in this way?

DR. YU   The characteristic symptoms of whooping cough, which manifest during the paroxysmal (spasmodic) phase, include a persistent, spasmodic, hacking cough with long gasps for air that create the characteristic whooping sound. When extreme, coughing may induce vomiting, nosebleeds, or bleeding from the eyes. Such symptoms are clear indications that Lung/metal has been severely damaged, causing the drying out of thick and fine fluids, and ascent of phlegm-fire. So, what exactly is this pathogenic qi that is relentlessly surging upward? Another way to ask the question might be, in the human body, what type of pathogenic qi could have such an intense, ascendant, and surging force? I am afraid that only Liver qi and Liver fire can wreak such havoc.

The reason for this is that perverse, rebellious, violent ascent of Liver qi can bring about Liver fire, which irrepressibly flares upward (a surplus of qi becomes fire). We can compare this idea with what we know from the *Classic of Changes (Yì jīng)*. Liver belongs to wood, and the trigram that represents that aspect is ☳ 'thunder' (震 *zhèn*). Hence, ministerial fire stored in the Liver is called 'thunder fire.' As its force is so formidable, it is also called 'thunderbolt fire' (霹靂火 *pī lì huǒ*). This Liver fire can counter-insult or rebel against Lung/metal. In Chinese medicine this is called 'wood fire punishing metal,' or, expressed differently, Liver fire punishing the Lung.

Delving deeper into this analogy, the idea is that this 'thunder fire' normally rests quietly, deep within Liver/wood. The question is, what has caused it to float to the exterior and to so aggressively ascend? My thinking is that it may have been because the whooping cough bacteria possesses an intense scorching nature that severely consumes the true yin of the Liver and Kidneys. This is based on the principle that the Liver and Kidneys have the same origin and when Liver yin is damaged, Kidney yin is usually damaged even more. When Kidney yin is damaged, water cannot nourish wood, which further exacerbates damage to Liver yin. When the yin of the Liver and Kidneys is damaged, then the thunder fire stored within the Liver loses its source of nourishment and its ability to stay settled within the Liver. Inevitably, the thunder fire floats up and outward, oversteps its normal boundaries, and punishes Lung/metal. I will leave it to all of you to further explore the issue of whether I am justified in using the phrase "toxicity damaging the Liver and Kidneys with Liver fire punishing the Lung" to describe the pathodynamic involved in this case.

PHYSICIAN C   If the pattern in this case is Liver fire rising uncontrollably, the treatment principle should be to use a large dosage of herbs that clear Liver and drain fire. The formula you use in this case, however, does not follow this line of reasoning.

DR. YU   There are two types of Liver fire: excess fire and deficiency fire. The term 'thunder fire' used as a description of Liver fire primarily refers to deficiency fire. Suitable treatment should enrich and nourish to contain and subdue thunder fire. In the metaphor of court officials found in Chapter 8 of the *Basic Questions (Sù wèn)*, the Liver is seen as the general. Its nature is harsh and aggressive. Even when excess fire is part of a Liver condition, it is inappropriate to use a large dosage of cold, bitter herbs. Cold, bitter herbs dry things out, are drying in nature and further damage Liver yin, which then causes Liver fire to ascend out of control even more strongly.

Whenever treating this type of pattern, I keep in mind what I learned from my teacher. Keep the treatment focused on following the principle of enriching and nourishing Liver yin while restraining thunder fire. Herbs to nourish Liver yin and restrain thunder fire are combined with medicinal substances to enrich the Kidneys, resolve toxicity, moisten the Lung, and dislodge phlegm. I customarily use a modification of Master Jian's Whooping Cough Formula *(Jiǎn shì dùn ké fāng)*.

The combination of Paeoniae Radix alba *(bái sháo)* and Glycyrrhizae Radix *(gān cǎo)* with Pheretima *(dì lóng)*, Cicadae Periostracum *(chán tuì)*, and Coptidis Rhizoma *(huáng lián)* acts to nourish the Liver and restrain fire. Scrophulariae Radix *(xuán shēn)*, Ophiopogonis Radix *(mài mén dōng)*, and Ostreae Concha *(mǔ lì)* are combined with Woodwardiae Rhizoma *(gǒu jǐ guàn zhòng)* and Bombyx batryticatus *(bái jiāng cán)* to enrich the Kidneys and resolve toxicity. Glehniae Radix *(běi shā shēn)* and Ophiopogonis Radix *(mài mén dōng)* combine with artificial Bambusae Concretio silicea *(rén gōng tiān zhú huáng)* to moisten the Lung and dislodge phlegm. The formula also contains Three Bugs Decoction *(sān chóng tāng)*—Bombyx batryticatus *(bái jiāng cán)*, Pheretima *(dì lóng)* and Cicadae Periostracum *(chán tuì)*—which, when combined with powdered Scolopendra *(wú gōng)* and Glycyrrhizae Radix *(gān cǎo)*, has a powerful ability to relieve spasms and unblock the collaterals. Thus the formula is reliably effective.

PHYSICIAN B Dr. Yu, the version of Master Jian's Whooping Cough Formula *(Jiǎn shì dùn ké fāng)* you gave the patient was modified. May I ask, what herbs make up the original formula?

DR. YU The original formula was created by my teacher, Jian Yu-Guang, who used it to treat the paroxysmal phase of whooping cough. It consists of six ingredients:

Paeoniae Radix alba *(bái sháo)*	15g
Ophiopogonis Radix *(mài mén dōng)*	15g
Scrophulariae Radix *(xuán shēn)*	15g
Schisandrae Fructus *(wǔ wèi zǐ)*	6g
Ostreae Concha *(mǔ lì)*	30g
Woodwardiae Rhizoma *(gǒu jǐ guàn zhòng)*	15g

Dr. Jian developed the formula during the latter half of the 1960s when, for several years, whooping cough was quite prevalent in the villages near Chengdu during the winter and spring. Many people had tried patent medicines and single-herb folk medicines to treat the symptoms of whooping cough's paroxysmal phase, but results were poor.

Master Jian used Paeoniae Radix alba *(bái sháo)* and Schisandrae Fructus *(wǔ wèi zǐ)* to nourish Liver yin, Ophiopogonis Radix *(mài mén dōng)* to moisten Lung dryness, Scrophulariae Radix *(xuán shēn)*, Ostreae Concha *(mǔ lì)*, and Woodwardiae Rhizoma *(gǒu jǐ guàn zhòng)* to enrich the Kidneys and resolve toxicity. The medicinal substances in the formula seem ordinary, but when modified with other herbs to address specific symptoms, the combination is able to quickly alleviate the symptoms of spasmodic cough. If I hadn't seen it work with my own eyes, I would never have believed it.

There are a few specific modifications that can be made to the formula. With fever, add Artemisiae annuae Herba *(qīng hāo)* and Gypsum fibrosum *(shí gāo)*. With the coughing up of blood or nosebleeds, add Platycladi Cacumen *(cè bǎi yè)*[12] and Imperatae Rhizoma *(bái máo gēn)*. If the patient has red eyes or is bleeding from the eyes, add Equiseti hiemalis Herba *(mù zéi)* and Buddlejae Flos *(mì měng huā)*. For vomiting, add Bambusae Caulis in taeniam *(zhú rú)* and unprocessed Haematitum *(shēng dài zhě shí)*. If, after taking two packets of the formula the effects aren't particularly obvious, combine the formula with 1.5g of a ground mixture of Bombyx batryticatus *(bái jiāng cán)*, Scolopendra *(wú gōng)*, Pheretima *(dì lóng)*, and Cicadae Periostracum *(chán tuì)* combined with honey water and taken three times a day. Master Jian once said that the paroxysmal (spasmodic) phase of whooping cough is usually due to damage to the true yin of the Liver, Lung, and Kidneys, which then leads to ascent of uncontrolled Liver fire. Consequently, when modifying Master Jian's Whooping Cough Formula *(Jiǎn shì dùn ké fāng)*, avoid using substances that are bitter and cold or enriching and cloying, and use ones that uplift qi, are discharging and dispersing in nature. Following this advice will usually bring good results.

PHYSICIAN A   Is it possible that the substances in Master Jian's Whooping Cough Formula *(Jiǎn shì dùn ké fāng)* primarily responsible for such good results are Bombyx batryticatus *(bái jiāng cán)*, Pheretima *(dì lóng)*, and Cicadae Periostracum *(chán tuì)*?

DR. YU   The ability of bugs to discharge heat, extinguish wind, resolve spasms, and suppress cough is far superior to those of plant-based substances. There are two contemporary doctors who are famous for their use of medicinal bugs, Zhang Ci-Gong and his student Zhu Liang-Chun. Zhu recommends three bug-based experiential formulas for treating whooping cough. I have tried each of them individually and have found them to be quite effective. In addition to the powdered Scolopendra *(wú gōng)* and Glycyrrhizae Radix *(gān cǎo)* combination that I used in this case, there are two others:

1. Paroxysmal Cough Powder *(dùn ké sǎn)*: Use 6g each of Cicadae Periostracum *(chán tuì)*, Bombyx batryticatus *(bái jiāng cán)*, and Peucedani Radix *(qián hú)* with 4.5g each of Gypsum fibrosum *(shí gāo)*, Armeniacae Semen *(xìng rén)*, Fritillariae cirrhosae Bulbus *(chuān bèi mǔ)*, and Costaziae Os *(fú hǎi shí)* and 1.5g each of Rhododendri Mollis Fructus *(liù zhóu zǐ)*,[13] Asari Radix et Rhizoma *(xì xīn)*, and Arisaema cum Bile *(chén jīng dǎn)*. The ingredients should be ground together into a very fine powder and a dose of 0.3g times the age of the patient is to be taken each time. This dosage can be taken 4-5 times each day (at least three hours apart) with boiled water sweetened with sugar.

....

12. *Translators' note:* The original text called for Cupressus funebris *(bó shù guǒ)*, which stops bleeding and quiets the spirit. Because this substance is not commonly available in the West, Dr. Yu suggested the above as a substitute.

13. Rhododendri Mollis Fructus (六軸子 *liù zhóu zǐ*) is bitter, warm, and has some toxicity. It dispels wind, dries dampness, disperses stasis, stops pain, calms wheezing, and stops diarrhea. Most commonly it is ground into a powder with 0.1 - 0.3g ingested per dose.

2. Wasp Nest and Rock Sugar Solution *(fáng fēng bīng tang yè)*: Take one entire Vespae Nidus nest *(lù fēng fáng)*, pour boiling water over it to steep, four to five times, until the water stops turning red. After this, use fresh water to rinse the nest a few times. Wrap the nest in gauze or cheese cloth, add two cups of water, and boil briefly. Add 50g of rock sugar and cook until the sugar is completely dissolved. The patient should drink the entire decoction once it has cooled down.

Because there are some challenges to making Paroxysmal Cough Powder *(dùn ké sǎn)*, I usually just add Scolopendra *(wú gōng)* and Glycyrrhizae Radix *(gān cǎo)* powder or Wasp Nest and Rock Sugar Solution *(fēng fáng bīng tang yè)* to Master Jian's Whooping Cough Formula *(Jiǎn shì dùn ké fāng)*.

CHAPTER 5

Disorders of the Eyes, Ears, Nose and Throat

5.1.1 Throat and oral cavity

CASE 1: Chronic pharyngitis (painful obstruction of the throat)

Why such minimal results?

收效甚微爲什麼?

■ CASE HISTORY

Patient: *38-year-old female*

Over the past three years this patient experienced multiple occurrences of her throat becoming dry, rough, irritated, and mildly painful, with a slight burning sensation. This was accompanied by the feeling of an object in the throat that could neither be swallowed nor expectorated. She also sporadically experienced a dry cough and hoarseness. Symptoms were mild in the morning and became more severe in the afternoon and evening.

The patient's biomedical diagnosis was chronic pharyngitis for which she had been prescribed antibiotics. After these proved ineffective, a steroid (prednisone) was added and some improvement followed. However, once these medicines were discontinued the symptoms returned, worse than before. The patient was therefore unwilling to retry this regime. This was followed by two rounds of cryotherapy that brought some relief. When the patient subsequently caught a cold, however, the symptoms returned.

She received a Chinese medical diagnosis of deficiency fire painful obstruction of the throat owing to exhaustion of Lung and Kidney yin with ascendant flaring of deficiency fire.

This led to her being prescribed more than 30 packets of formulas like Lily Bulb Decoction to Preserve the Metal *(bǎi hé gù jīn tāng)*, Anemarrhena, Phellodendron, and Rehmannia Pill *(zhī bǎi dì huáng wán)* and Nourish the Yin and Clear the Lung Decoction *(yǎng yīn qīng fèi tāng)*. While this line of treatment mitigated the symptoms, it also caused the patient to eat less and develop a cold feeling in her abdomen.

Treatment was then directed at a diagnosis of plum-pit qi for which three packets of a combination of Pinellia and Magnolia Bark Decoction *(bàn xià hòu pò tāng)* and Augmented Rambling Powder *(jiā wèi xiāo yáo sǎn)* was prescribed. This led to an increase in the dryness and burning sensation in her throat. Having endured this condition for three years, the patient lost confidence in treatment.

INTAKE EXAMINATION
DATE: May 23, 1992

The disorder was as described above and included a slightly dry mouth with a bland taste in the mouth and an inability to taste food, sub-par food intake, and stools that tended toward dryness. The woman's menstrual blood was copious and tended to be pale. Examination of the pharynx revealed that the mucous membranes were pale red and slightly dry. Clusters of lymphofollicular hyperplasia had formed on the posterior wall of the pharynx. The patient's tongue was pale with scant moisture and a thin, white coating. Her pulse was moderate and weak.

DIFFERENTIATION OF PATTERN AND DISCUSSION OF TREATMENT

PHYSICIAN A   The standard Chinese medicine textbooks say that chronic pharyngitis is equivalent to deficiency fire painful obstruction of the throat, and that the important diagnostic parameters are discomfort in the throat, slight pain, feeling of an object in the throat, and frequent throat clearing. Examination of the pharynx should reveal slight redness and small spots of hyperplasia at the base of the throat. Since the case at hand thoroughly fits this picture, why do we not proceed with treatment that corresponds to this diagnosis?

DR. YU   This case is not one of Lung and Kidney yin deficiency.

Let us investigate evidence of symptoms that relate to ascendant flaring of deficiency fire:

• The pharyngeal membrane is pale red, not slightly dark red. Also, the observed lymphofollicular hyperplasia was massive instead of granular. The tongue is pale red with scant moisture, the pulse is moderate and weak, not rapid. There are no indications of ascendant flaring of deficiency fire.

• The patient presents with a mouth that is slightly dry with a diminished sense of taste, sub-par food intake, stools that are relatively dry, and menstrual blood that is rather copious and tends to be pale. From this we can consider a pattern of Spleen yin exhaustion along with insufficiency of Spleen qi.

The patient had already taken dozens of packets of formulas that nourish yin and direct fire downward. This led to only limited improvement along with some undesirable side effects, so we should not go down that road again.

TREATMENT AND OUTCOME

The Spleen and Stomach pertain to earth. Earth organ disorders require sweet and moderate herbs. Furthermore, to nourish and enrich Spleen yin it is particularly suitable to rely mainly on sweet, bland, and moderate herbs or sweet, cool, moistening herbs and assist them with sweet, warm, tonifying substances to strengthen the Spleen and augment qi.

It is my custom to use a modification of Harmonize the Six Decoction *(liù hé tāng)*, a formula from the Ming-dynasty work *Five Texts by [Hu] Shen-Rou (Shèn-Róu wǔ shū)* that nourishes and enriches Spleen yin, or to modify Ginseng, Poria, and White Atractylodes Powder *(shēn líng bái zhú sǎn)* by removing the acrid and drying herbs and adding sweet, cool, and moistening ones.

Consider this to be a pattern of Spleen yin exhaustion that causes loss of nourishment and moisture in the throat. Treatment then can aim to enrich and nourish Spleen yin and augment Spleen qi. When the Spleen yin and qi are ample, they continuously rise to the throat and its surrounding area.

Formula 1: Modification of Harmonize the Six Decoction *(liù hé tāng)*

Pseudostellariae Radix *(tài zǐ shēn)*	15g
Hordei Fructus germinatus *(mài yá)*	15g
Poria *(fú líng)*	12g
Glycyrrhizae Radix *(gān cǎo)*	5g
Glycyrrhizae Radix praeparata *(zhì gān cǎo)*	5g
untreated Lablab Semen album *(shēng bái biǎn dòu)*	15g
Dioscoreae Rhizoma *(shān yào)*	20g
Lilii Bulbus *(bǎi hé)*	30g
Astragali Radix *(huáng qí)*	20g
Platycodi Radix *(jié gěng)*	10g
Oroxyli Semen *(mù hú dié)*	10g

Instructions: Six packets were prescribed, cooked as a decoction, and each packet divided into three daily doses.

Formula 2: Experiential formula from Zhang Xi-Chun

Mori Folium *(sāng yè)*	6g
Menthae haplocalycis Herba *(bò hé)*	6g
Talcum *(huá shí)*	30g
Glycyrrhizae Radix *(gān cǎo)*	6g
Cicadae Periostracum *(chán tuì)*	6g
Sterculiae lychnophorae Semen *(pàng dà hǎi)*	3 pieces
Ophiopogonis Radix *(mài mén dōng)*	15g

Instructions: Six packets were prescribed. To be steeped in boiled water and drunk throughout the day as a tea.

SECOND VISIT: The patient's sensation of dryness, roughness, and various symptoms of discomfort in her throat had diminished. Her appetite had improved, and her mouth was no longer dry. Bowel movements were now smooth.

The formula was changed to a modified combination of Harmonize the Six Decoction *(liù hé tāng)* and Ginseng, Poria, and White Atractylodes Powder *(shēn líng bái zhú sǎn)* as follows:

Pseudostellariae Radix *(tài zǐ shēn)* 50g
Atractylodis macrocephalae Rhizoma *(bái zhú)* 30g
Poria *(fú líng)* 30g
Glycyrrhizae Radix *(gān cǎo)* 15g
Glycyrrhizae Radix praeparata *(zhì gān cǎo)* 15g
untreated Lablab Semen album *(shēng bái biǎn dòu)* 30g
Dioscoreae Rhizoma *(shān yào)* 50g
Lilii Bulbus *(bǎi hé)* 100g
Astragali Radix *(huáng qí)* 60g
Platycodi Radix *(jié gěng)* 15g
Oroxyli Semen *(mù hú dié)* 30g
golden hairpin Dendrobii Herba *(jīn chāishí hú)* 50g
Nelumbinis Semen *(lián zǐ)* (center removed) 50g
Vespae Nidus *(lù fēng fáng)* 20g
Curcumae Radix *(yù jīn)* 30g
Albiziae Flos *(hé huān huā)* 30g
Fritillariae thunbergii Bulbus *(zhè bèi mǔ)* 50g

METHOD OF PREPARATION: The herbs were gently roasted until crisp and then ground to a powder. The powder was mixed with refined honey to make pills. Each pill should weigh 10g.

The patient was instructed to take one pill, three times per day, and continue this regimen for one month.

OUTCOME: After taking one course of this formula the patient's symptoms of dry and rough throat, slight pain, burning sensation, and feeling of an object in the throat had all diminished in severity. At times her throat felt normal. The patient then prepared and took another course of the formula after which the symptoms completely receded and her voice became clear. Upon examination, her pharyngeal membranes were red and moist, and the posterior wall of the pharynx was smooth with no sign of lymphofollicular hyperplasia. Over the course of the following two years the patient came down with a cold or flu three times with no recurrence of pharyngitis.

Whenever occasional throat discomfort occurred it was treated successfully with one or two packets of Six Ingredient Decoction *(liù wèi tāng)*—Schizonepetae Herba *(jīng jiè)*, Saposhnikoviae Radix *(fáng fēng)*, Platycodi Radix *(jié gěng)*, Glycyrrhizae Radix *(gān cǎo)*, Bombyx batryticatus *(bái jiāng cán)* and Menthae haplocalycis Herba *(bò hé)*.

Disease	Primary symptoms	Differential diagnosis	Treatment method	Formula
Chronic pharyngitis	Dry and slightly painful pharynx, burning sensation, feeling of an object in the throat	Spleen yin exhaustion leaving the pharynx without moisture and nourishment	Enrich and nourish the Spleen yin and augment Spleen qi	Harmonize the Six Decoction *(liù hé tāng)*

DR. YU   In the past we have discussed deficiency cold pharyngitis and chronic pharyngitis that can cause a laryngeal cough. Today we want to talk about pattern differentiation and treatment of chronic pharyngitis that arises from Spleen yin exhaustion. This pattern is commonly seen in practice and today's case is a good example. It is worth noting that a not small number of practitioners categorize and treat this disorder as Lung and Kidney deficiency with upward blazing of deficiency fire, and with only minimal benefit.

PHYSICIAN B   Dr. Yu, despite there being no precedent for this in the literature, you place emphasis on approaching discussion and treatment of chronic pharyngitis from the viewpoint of the Spleen and Stomach. Do you have some special understanding of this?

DR. YU   The pharynx is in the back of the throat. Through the esophagus below, it connects directly to the stomach. In Chapter 69 of the *Divine Pivot (Líng shū)* it states that "the pharynx and throat are the path of liquids and grain" while in Chapter 29 of the *Basic Question (Sū wèn)* it says that "the pharynx governs earth qi." From this we can see that the pharynx is under the province of the Spleen-Stomach, and disease processes of the pharynx have an intimate relationship with these organs. This is easy to comprehend.

From a clinical perspective, it is completely accurate to say that chronic pharyngitis is often due to Spleen yin exhaustion or a loss of the Spleen's capacity to transport. This is especially true in middle-aged women. However, most modern texts categorize this disorder as one of deficiency fire painful obstruction of the throat and treat it as blazing ascent of deficiency fire from Lung and Kidney yin deficiency. This leads to treatment with formulas such as Six-Ingredient Pill with Rehmannia *(liù wèi dì huáng wán)* and Anemarrhena, Phellodendron, and Rehmannia Pill *(zhī bǎi dì huáng wán)* and poor outcomes where the symptoms often worsen. It may be worthwhile to reconsider this categorization.

As we have discussed previously, patients who have Spleen-Stomach type chronic pharyngitis usually do not have symptoms of blazing ascent of deficiency fire in the pharynx or the rest of the body and do not display a pulse and tongue that correspond with that pattern. This type of patient generally has a dry pharynx, but not a dry mouth, a tongue that is of normal color or tending to pale, and a pulse that is weak or soggy. Not infrequently, this patient will have disorders of the gastrointestinal tract such as chronic superficial gastritis, peptic ulcer, or functional gastrointestinal tract dysfunction. Therefore, the pattern mainly involves the Spleen-Stomach and not the Lung-Kidney. If we understand this logic there is no need to overthink: we know that the pharynx is the gate to the Spleen-Stomach and from this we can deduce the rest.

PHYSICIAN C   But in the clinic we certainly see cases of chronic pharyngitis resulting from Lung-Kidney yin deficiency with blazing ascent of deficiency fire.

DR. YU   Surely, this is frequently seen in men who over-indulge in tobacco and alcohol. If treatment of this pattern uses Anemarrhena, Phellodendron, and Rehmannia Pill *(zhī bǎi dì huáng wán)* or Nourish the Yin and Clear the Lung Decoction *(yǎng yīn qīng fèi tāng)* and the results are unsatisfactory, one can try improving efficacy by using Special Pill for the Three Talents that Seals the Marrow *(sān cái fēng suǐ dān)* from the 12th-century text, *Formulas to Protect Life and the Most Treasured Family Possession*

(Wèi shēng jiā bǎo fāng)—Asparagi Radix *(tiān mén dōng)*, Rehmanniae Radix *(shēng dì huáng)*, Ginseng Radix *(rén shēn)* (substitute Glehniae/Adenophorae Radix *[shā shēn]*), Amomi Fructus *(shā rén)*, Phellodendri Cortex *(huáng bǎi)*, and Glycyrrhizae Radix *(gān cǎo)*—and modifying the formula according to the presenting pattern.

PHYSICIAN C   Mild cases of chronic pharyngitis are not difficult to treat. What is difficult is eliminating lymphofollicular hyperplasia.

DR. YU   It is difficult to eliminate that in the short term. Formula books suggest adding herbs such as Platycodi Radix *(jié gěng)*, Cyperi Rhizoma *(xiāng fù)*, Curcumae Radix *(yù jīn)*, and Albiziae Flos *(hé huān huā)* to move qi, invigorate blood, relieve constraint, and dissipate knots. It is my habit to use herbs such as Fritillariae thunbergii Bulbus *(zhè bèi mǔ)*, Vespae Nidus *(lù fēng fáng)*, Ostreae Concha *(mǔ lì)*, and Curcumae Radix *(yù jīn)*. I have found these to be slightly more effective.

PHYSICIAN A   How do we approach treatment of chronic pharyngitis that is part of a pattern of Spleen losing its capacity to transport?

DR. YU   In addition to inflammation of the pharynx, chronic pharyngitis that is part of a pattern of Spleen losing its capacity to transport is often accompanied by other indications of that pattern. These include symptoms such as copious oral mucus, nausea while brushing one's teeth upon arising in the morning, or gastric cavity focal distention and abdominal distention with intestinal rumbling and watery stools. Treatment should center on augmenting and moving Spleen qi with Six-Gentlemen Decoction with Aucklandia and Amomum *(xiāng shā liù jūn zǐ tāng)* modified by adding herbs such as Platycodi Radix *(jié gěng)*, Oroxyli Semen *(mù hú dié)*, and Kaki Calyx *(shì dì)*.

- If the pattern includes Liver constraint with mood swings and discomfort in the chest and lateral costal region, add Bupleuri Radix *(chái hú)* and Tribuli Fructus *(cì jí lí)*.

- For intestinal rumbling and diarrhea, add Zingiberis Rhizoma praeparatum *(páo jiāng)* and Agrimoniae Herba *(xiān hè cǎo)*.

- For dizziness, add Alismatis Rhizoma *(zé xiè)*.

- For Spleen deficiency that extends to the Heart and gives rise to fright palpitations and lack of sleep, first use several packets of Restore the Spleen Decoction *(guī pí tāng)* with standard Pinelliae Rhizoma praeparatum *(fǎ bàn xià)* and Prunellae Spica *(xià kū cǎo)* and then switch to Six-Gentlemen Decoction with Aucklandia and Amomum *(xiāng shā liù jūn zǐ tāng)*.

- If the qi is exhausted to the extent of exhausting the yang, manifesting as copious and clear, thin secretions in the throat, loose stools and a fear of cold, this is classified as deficiency cold pharyngitis for which we should use formulas that warm and tonify the Spleen and Kidney. This is something we will discuss in the next case, so we will not address it here.

PHYSICIAN B   Nowadays there are those who feel that discussion and treatment of chronic pharyngitis falls within the scope of plum-pit qi. Do you think that is correct?

DR. YU   Plum-pit qi should encompass a portion of cases of chronic pharyngitis. When ancient texts discuss plum-pit qi they pay careful attention to the feeling—with or without basis—of something in the pharyngeal area of the throat (the semblance of something obstructing the pharynx and this something cannot be coughed up or swallowed down). Modern biomedical texts have mimicked this categorization by defining cases of plum-pit qi where examination of the pharyngeal area reveals nothing unusual, as in pharyngeal neurosis or globus hystericus. In the clinic, a portion of the cases of chronic pharyngitis that we see display very slight abnormalities of the pharynx (such as chronic hyperemia or lymphofollicular hyperplasia in the posterior wall of the pharynx), but the main symptom is a feeling of something in the throat or a tightness in the throat which is often exacerbated by changes in mood. I feel that this type of chronic pharyngitis can rightly be treated as plum-pit qi.

PHYSICIAN A   Dr. Yu, are you saying that this type of chronic pharyngitis can be treated with Pinellia and Magnolia Bark Decoction *(bàn xià hòu pò tāng)*?

DR. YU   In the *Essentials from the Golden Cabinet (Jīn guì yào lüè)*, Pinellia and Magnolia Bark Decoction *(bàn xià hòu pò tāng)* treats plum-pit qi that is the outcome of stagnant obstruction of phlegm and qi. For this it is definitely effective. However, if the patient's pattern is not one of stagnant obstruction of phlegm, or if the patient also suffers from injury to yin, this formula is not appropriate.

As an example, in 1984 I treated a 35-year-old unmarried woman who was weighed down with stress and worry. She had a reduced appetite, confused dreams, and irregular menstruation. For the previous three months she had experienced an uncomfortable feeling of obstruction in her throat that could neither be swallowed nor spit up. She had been examined in the ear, nose, and throat department and found to have a small measure of lymphofollicular hyperplasia. Her tongue was slightly red with a thin, yellow coating and her pulse was wiry and fine.

She was given Pinellia and Magnolia Bark Decoction *(bàn xià hòu pò tāng)* with the addition of Ziziphi spinosae Semen *(suān zǎo rén)*, Platycodi Radix *(jié gěng)*, Inulae Flos *(xuán fù huā)*, and Glycyrrhizae Radix *(gān cǎo)*. After one packet her throat and nose were dry. She took one more packet and experienced burning pain in her stomach, irritability, and an aggravated sense of there being an object in her throat.

Reassessment of the formula revealed that we had not considered the possibility that long-term Liver constraint had transformed into fire and damaged the yin. We had also ignored the clues that would have revealed this, for instance, a wiry and fine pulse and a red tongue with a thin, yellow coating.

Consequently, we changed our treatment to one using Clear the Liver Drink *(qīng gān yǐn)* and Two-Solstice Pill *(èr zhì wán)* to enrich water and clear the Liver. After two packets there was slight relief. The formula was modified according to presenting symptoms and 36 packets were taken in total. The patient's feeling that there was an object in her throat completely receded. This leads us to remember the famous Qing-dynasty physician Wu Ju-Tong who stated that, when wishing to dispense an effective formula we should wholly rely on "recognizing the pattern without error," and of Pu Fu-Zhou who urged us to achieve "one formula for each person." When prescribing herbs, we should heed the experience on which these statements are based and pay attention to each person's unique situation.

5.1.2 **Throat and oral cavity**

CASE 2: **Six months of pharyngeal pain**

The strategic move of using a testing formula

舉棋難定的 "試探法"

■ CASE HISTORY

Patient: *10-year-old boy*

Six months previously the patient came down with an externally-contracted disorder marked by a swollen and painful throat, high fever, and a productive cough with thick, yellow phlegm. He was in the hospital for one week and the disorder resolved. His swollen and painful throat was almost completely better, with only a bit of pain remaining. Since then, however, the condition has continued to come and go. Whenever he would contract a mild external disorder, his throat pain would worsen and be accompanied by a cough with phlegm that was difficult to expectorate along with hoarseness.

Because the patient had repeatedly tried antibiotics, anti-inflammatory drugs and intravenous drips as well as Chinese patent medicines such as Six-Miracle Pill *(liù shén wán)* and Isatis Root Granules *(bǎn lán gēn chōng jī)* without success, the family decided to try Chinese herbs. The doctors diagnosed the boy as having uncleared residual heat in the upper burner and prescribed herbs to dredge wind, clear heat, resolve toxicity and disperse knots. Treatment included over 20 packets in total of formulas like Forsythia and Mentha Decoction *(qiáo hé tāng)*, Honeysuckle, Forsythia, and Puffball Powder *(yín qiáo mǎ bó sǎn)*, and Clear the Throat and Enable the Diaphragm Decoction *(qīng yān lì gé tāng)*. Not only did the throat pain fail to diminish, the patient also experienced reduced food intake and loose stools.

Another doctor thought that the diagnosis of uncleared residual heat in the upper burner was correct, but because this was a chronic disorder the herbs should be taken in powdered form. Thus, the herbs of Forsythia and Mentha Decoction *(qiáo hé tāng)*, Honeysuckle, Forsythia, and Puffball Powder *(yín qiáo mǎ bó sǎn)* and Clear the Throat and Enable the Diaphragm Decoction *(qīng yān lì gé tāng)* were roasted and ground to a powder and the patient took the powder for more than one month. His throat pain remained unchanged.

The child's mother was at a loss and so brought him to our clinic for treatment.

INTAKE EXAMINATION
DATE: April 4, 1990

The patient's throat was itchy and slightly sore and he had a cough that produced sticky, white phlegm. He had a hoarse voice, reduced food intake, and loose stools. His complexion lacked luster, his pharyngeal area was pale white and had a spot of ball-shaped hyperplasia. The right side of his tonsils had two areas, each the size of a soybean, covered with yellow-white pus-filled depressions. His tongue was pale red with a thin, white coating, and his pulse was moderate and weak.

DIFFERENTIATION OF PATTERN AND DISCUSSION OF TREATMENT

PHYSICIAN A   Conventional wisdom is that "throat disorders all belong to fire," be it excess fire or deficiency fire. But in the present case, the chronic pharyngitis and tonsillitis caused only slight pain. After repeated use of antibiotics, anti-inflammatories and intravenous drugs were ineffective, Chinese medicines that dredge wind, clear heat, resolve toxicity, unblock the throat and nourish yin, lead fire downward and return fire to its source also failed to be effective. Treatment dragged on for half a year. These things illustrate that this case is neither excess fire nor deficiency fire.

DR. YU   In my early years of treating chronic pharyngitis I strictly followed the concept expressed in the maxim, "throat disorders all belong to fire," and I used acrid and cool herbs to disperse wind, bitter and cold herbs to clear heat, and sweet and cold herbs to nourish yin. This was sometimes effective and sometimes not. In cases where this was ineffective, I still did not dare to use warm or hot herbs.

Later, when I was working in Chengdu, I saw an old Chinese doctor frequently treat chronic pharyngitis with Cinnamon Twig Decoction *(guì zhī tāng)* with the addition of Zingiberis Rhizoma *(gān jiāng)*. I saw another old Chinese doctor frequently use Ephedra, Asarum, and Aconite Accessory Root Decoction *(má huáng xì xīn fù zǐ tāng)* for this condition. Though they were questioned about the wisdom of this by their patients, they did not change their ways. Despite the negative feedback, there were also a sizable number of reports of effective results. I now believe that if you want to treat this disorder you must not abandon warm and hot herbs. Over time and after careful analysis of treatments, I began to understand that chronic pharyngitis is often the result of deficiency fire. When cold and cool herbs are used, the situation can drag on and gradually damage both the yin and yang and transform into a deficiency-cold pattern. This is especially true if the patient has a yang-deficient constitution and repeatedly contracts wind-cold pathogens.

I have examined many deficiency-cold pharyngitis patients; again and again their throats had granular hyperplasia, slight pain, and a feeling of a foreign body in the throat. Although this closely mimics deficiency-fire pharyngitis, in these patients the symptoms are also frequently accompanied by some symptoms of deficiency-cold such as clear, thin, fishy-smelling and copious secretions in the throat, a dry throat without a dry mouth, clear, copious urine, loose stools, fear of cold and susceptibility to catching cold. The tongue of these patients is pale or pale purple with a coating that is white and moist, white and greasy, slightly yellow with plentiful fluids, or black and moist. These patients have a pulse that is moderate and weak or submerged and weak. Furthermore, this type of patient has repeatedly used antibiotics or cold and cooling herbs. This does not have a positive effect, and in fact worsens the condition.

In the clinic, if one carefully inquires and pays close attention to the four examinations, it will not be difficult to recognize this pattern.

The pathogenesis of this disorder is Spleen deficiency and Lung cold with phlegm stagnating in the throat, or yang deficiency of the Spleen, Lung and Kidney with yin-cold congealed in the throat. Treatment of the former pattern is discussed in this case. For the latter pattern, one should warm yang, direct counterflow qi downward, dispel cold and free the throat from stagnation.

I have combined several classic formulas and named the combination Decoction for Deficiency-Cold Throat Painful Obstruction (xū hán hóu bì tāng):

standard Pinelliae Rhizoma praeparatum (fǎ bàn xià) 10g
Cinnamomi Ramulus (guì zhī) 10g
Glycyrrhizae Radix praeparata (zhì gān cǎo) 10g
Platycodi Radix (jié gěng) 10g
Codonopsis Radix (dǎng shēn) 15g
Atractylodis macrocephalae Rhizoma (bái zhú) 12g
Zingiberis Rhizoma praeparatum (páo jiāng) 6g
Aconiti Radix lateralis praeparata (zhì fù zǐ) 6g
Poria (fú líng) 15g

This formula contains Pinellia Powder or Decoction (bàn xià sǎn jí tāng), Licorice and Ginger Decoction (gān cǎo gān jiāng tāng), and Aconite Accessory Root Pill to Regulate the Middle (fù zǐ lǐ zhōng wán). Together these formulas warm yang, direct counterflow qi downward, dispel cold and free stagnation in the throat. I have used this formula to treat several dozens of cases and the results have been quite satisfactory.

Before using this formula, one must overcome two obstacles:

- First, there are cases where a deficiency-cold pattern is not very obvious and that makes one fearful of giving an incorrect formula.

- Second, although the practitioner may be certain that the patient fits the deficiency-cold pattern picture, the patient may be apprehensive about taking such hot herbs.

In either of these situations you can use a simplified version of Pinellia Powder or Decoction (bàn xià sǎn jí tāng) made up of standard Pinelliae Rhizoma praeparatum (fǎ bàn xià), Cinnamomi Ramulus (guì zhī), and Glycyrrhizae Radix (gān cǎo) (3g of each herb) as a testing formula. The cooking method for this formula is as follows:

Soak the herbs in about 130ml of room-temperature water for 15 minutes. Bring the mixture to a boil and simmer over a moderate flame for 15 minutes. After the herbs are strained out there should be about 100ml of liquid remaining. Have the patient take a small amount and let it linger in the throat before swallowing. Over the course of half a day the patient should finish the liquid.

If the patient does not really fit the deficiency-cold pattern picture, after drinking the decoction the feeling of discomfort in his or her throat will worsen. One should then quickly change the treatment approach. If the patient truly has deficiency-cold pharyngitis, they will feel their throat to be soothed by the decoction and there will be no side effects. At this time, I then feel free to prescribe Decoction for Deficiency-Cold Throat Painful Obstruction (xū hán hóu bì tāng); the patient's reservations are also eased by this test. I have had more and more of these cases and I have become quite convinced of this. Chronic pharyngitis is a complex and difficult condition to treat, but more difficult is overcoming the influence of the maxim, "throat disorders all belong to fire."

PHYSICIAN D   I heard long ago that when treating chronic pharyngitis you like to use warm and hot herbs like Zingiberis Rhizoma *(gān jiāng)*, Cinnamomi Ramulus *(guì zhī)* and Aconiti Radix lateralis praeparata *(zhì fù zǐ)*. How did you come to gain this insight? Can you share the trick to this with us?

DR. YU   It is not that I "like" to use warm and hot herbs for this condition, but rather that I specifically use them when treating deficiency-cold pharyngitis. This we have just discussed in detail.

PHYSICIAN E   Dr. Yu, if I could follow up on that with a question about the diagnosis of chronic pharyngitis that is due to deficiency-fire. You point out that this type of chronic pharyngitis should present with granular lymphofollicular hyperplasia rather than massive lymphofollicular hyperplasia. You also mention that chronic pharyngitis from deficiency-fire presents with a pharyngeal membrane that is slightly dark red. I have not heard of these diagnostic parameters. May I ask where they originate?

DR. YU   I learned of the diagnostic value of observing the back of the throat several years ago from some articles about the differential diagnosis of chronic pharyngitis. These practitioners observed that in cases that fit the pattern of deficiency-fire, the membranes at the back of the throat were dark red and slightly dry. They also noted that any lymphofollicular hyperplasia in patients with this pattern was generally granular. Since then, I have used a flashlight to observe the throats of patients with chronic pharyngitis.

TREATMENT AND OUTCOME

Consider this pattern as one of Spleen deficiency with Lung cold and phlegm stagnation in the throat. Treatment should promote proper movement by the Spleen (i.e., fortify the Spleen's capacity to transport), warm the Lung, transform phlegm, and free the throat of stagnation.

The main formula used in treatment is a melding of Six-Gentlemen Decoction with Aucklandia and Amomum *(xiāng shā liù jūn zǐ tāng)*, Poria, Cinnamon Twig, Atractylodes, and Licorice Decoction *(líng guì zhú gān tāng)*, and Licorice and Ginger Decoction *(gān cǎo gān jiāng tāng)* as follows:

Codonopsis Radix *(dǎng shēn)*	12g
Atractylodis macrocephalae Rhizoma *(bái zhú)*	10g
Poria *(fú líng)*	15g
Glycyrrhizae Radix praeparata *(zhì gān cǎo)*	5g
standard Pinelliae Rhizoma praeparatum *(fǎ bàn xià)*	12g
Citri reticulatae Pericarpium *(chén pí)*	10g
Amomi Fructus *(shā rén)*	[added near end] 5g
Aucklandiae Radix *(mù xiāng)*	10g
Zingiberis Rhizoma *(gān jiāng)*	6g
Zingiberis Rhizoma recens *(shēng jiāng)*	6g

Jujubae Fructus *(dà zǎo)* 10g
Cinnamomi Ramulus *(guì zhī)* 10g
Platycodi Radix *(jié gěng)* 10g

The patient's mother had some familiarity with Chinese medicine and was concerned with the warm herbs; she appeared worried. I said to her, "If you are afraid of the warmth of this formula you can first apply Musk and Tiger Bone Plaster *(shè xiāng hǔ gǔ gāo)*[1] to test the appropriateness of a warm formula." She got a patch and applied it to her son's neck. The following day the pharyngeal pain had decreased and so did her concern over using the warming formula.

OUTCOME

After three packets of herbs the patient's throat pain had ceased and the itching had greatly diminished. His cough had lessened, his food intake increased, and his stools were now well-formed. Examination of the patient's throat revealed that the pustules on his tonsils had disappeared.

We continued the above formula, removing Amomi Fructus *(shā rén)*, Aucklandiae Radix *(mù xiāng)*, Zingiberis Rhizoma recens *(shēng jiāng)*, and Jujubae Fructus *(dà zǎo)* while adding Fritillariae thunbergii Bulbus *(zhè bèi mǔ)* 10g, Oroxyli Semen *(mù hú dié)* 15g, Bombyx batryticatus *(bái jiāng cán)* 5g, and Vespae Nidus *(lù fēng fáng)* 6g. After he took six packets of this formula the patient's throat itching and cough were gone and his voice was clear. In addition, the patch of granular hyperplasia previously seen in his pharyngeal area was no longer present.

Disease	Primary symptoms	Differential diagnosis	Treatment method	Formula
Deficiency-cold pharyngitis	Itching and slight pain in the pharynx, reduced food intake and loose stools	Deficiency-cold in the Spleen and Lung, phlegm stagnation in the throat	Increase the Spleen's transporting function, warm the Lung, transform phlegm and unblock stagnation in the throat	A combination of Six-Gentlemen Decoction with Aucklandia and Amomum *(xiāng shā liù jūn zǐ tāng)*, Poria, Cinnamon Twig, Atractylodes, and Licorice Decoction *(líng guì zhú gān tāng)*, and Licorice and Ginger Decoction *(gān cǎo gān jiāng tāng)*

REFLECTIONS AND CLARIFICATIONS

PHYSICIAN B   Your viewpoint that this sore throat pattern is one of deficiency cold relies on two factors: first, that the disease process had persisted for six months, and second, that the extended use of antibiotics and anti-inflammatory drugs as well as herbs that clear heat, resolve toxicity along with those that enrich yin were all ineffective. Is this an accurate portrayal of your thinking?

....

1. *Translators' note:* While the listed ingredients in this plaster are not particularly hot, the unlisted ingredients include such very warm substances as Ephedrae Herba *(má huáng)*, Aconiti Radix praeparata *(zhì chuān wū)*, and Aconiti kusnezoffii Radix praeparata *(zhì cǎo wū)*. For the purposes noted here, any warming plaster will work.

DR. YU   We must also, as it states in line 16 of the *Discussion of Cold Damage (Shāng hán lùn)*, "[o]bserve their pulse and symptoms," as these are vital diagnostic pointers in our medicine. This child had itching and minor pain in his throat, but it was not red or swollen and there were no indications of heat. The granular hyperplasia was lumpy and pale white; this is characteristic of Spleen deficiency. The tonsils had both white and yellow pustules, but these were sunken and thus a sign of qi deficiency. Combining this information with indications such as a lusterless complexion, reduced food intake, loose stools, a pale tongue with a thin, white coating and a pulse that was moderate and weak, we can completely exclude the possibility of fire-heat or yin deficiency.

PHYSICIAN C   "The throat pertains to the Lung." Even though the pattern is one of deficiency cold it is also appropriate to focus on treating the Lung. What is the reason that you mainly use the Spleen-moving and phlegm-transforming Six-Gentlemen Decoction with Aucklandia and Amomum *(xiāng shā liù jūn zǐ tāng)*?

DR. YU   "The throat pertains to the Lung" is not precise. The ancients used the pairing of the characters for pharynx (咽 *yān*) and larynx (喉 *hóu*) to indicate the pharynx, and the term larynx-throat (喉嚨 *hóu lóng*) to indicate the larynx. Though they did not provide exact anatomical locations for these terms, they did recognize, as stated in Chapter 69 of the *Divine Pivot (Líng shū)*, that "The pharynx is the path of liquids and grains; the larynx is the place of ascent and descent of qi [air]." The fifth edition of the textbook *Traditional Chinese Otolaryngology (Zhōng yī ěr bí hóu kē xué)* clarifies the matter by stating that "The larynx is anterior, it links to the airway, connects to the Lung and belongs to the pulmonary system. The pharynx is posterior, it extends to the esophagus and belongs to the digestive system." Because of this it is easy to understand the use of Six-Gentlemen Decoction with Aucklandia and Amomum *(xiāng shā liù jūn zǐ tāng)* in this case of sore throat. This formula contains Four-Gentlemen Decoction *(sì jūn zǐ tāng)* to strengthen the Spleen and augment qi. As noted in the *Golden Mirror of the Medical Tradition (Yī zōng jīn jiàn)*:

> Citri reticulatae Pericarpium *(chén pí)* is added to facilitate [proper movement] of Lung-metal counterflow qi and Pinelliae Rhizoma praeparatum *(zhì bàn xià)* added to dredge the damp qi of Spleen-earth, so that phlegm and thin mucus are dispelled. Aucklandiae Radix *(mù xiāng)* is added to properly move qi that has stagnated in the Triple Burner and Amomi Fructus *(shā rén)* is added to unblock the basal qi of the Spleen and Kidneys, so that which is stuck and constrained (膹鬱 *fèn yù*)[2] can be unblocked.

We can see that this formula truly treats both the Spleen and Lung by "nurturing earth to engender metal." When paired with Poria, Cinnamon Twig, Atractylodes, and Licorice Decoction *(líng guì zhú gān tāng)* and Licorice and Ginger Decoction *(gān cǎo gān jiāng tāng)* to warm yang and transform thin mucus, it is even more suitable for treating the pathodynamic of Spleen-deficiency, Lung-cold phlegm stagnation in the throat.

PHYSICIAN B   Dr. Yu, upon considering your earlier failures, you made a radical shift to take a path less chosen by using Six-Gentlemen Decoction with Aucklandia and Amo-

....

2. *Translators' note:* This is a term from Chapter 74 of the *Basic Questions (Sū wèn)* where it described a type of difficult breathing where there is fullness and tightness in the chest and epigastrium along with rapid gasping for breath.

mum *(xiāng shā liù jūn zǐ tāng)* combined with Poria, Cinnamon Twig, Atractylodes, and Licorice Decoction *(líng guì zhú gān tāng)* and Licorice and Ginger Decoction *(gān cǎo gān jiāng tāng)* to move the Spleen qi and transform phlegm, warm the Lung and transform thin mucus. The success of this treatment demonstrates that this pharyngitis was correctly categorized as belonging to deficiency cold. Although this case is an exception, it provides a useful reference.

DR. YU   I will take issue with your choice of the word "exception" because that word implies something infrequent or rarely seen. In clinical work, this is not in fact the case. There are numerous references in classical literature that demonstrate our predecessors' treatment of deficiency-cold throat disorders using formulas that warm the channels, disperse cold, warm the middle and strengthen the Spleen, or formulas that warm yang and tonify the Kidneys. A prominent example is found in line 313 of the *Discussion of Cold Damage* where Pinellia Powder or Decoction *(bàn xià sǎn jí tāng)*[3] is cited for treatment of throat pain owing to cold lodged in the *shào yīn*.

PHYSICIAN B   But, after all, the concept of "throat disorders all belong to fire" originates in Chapter 7 of the *Basic Questions (Sū wèn)* where it states that the "knotting of one yin and one yang is referred to as throat obstruction." How do you interpret this?

DR. YU   I believe that the phrase "knotting of one yin and one yang is called throat obstruction" refers to throat disorders that are part of a pathodynamic where *jué yīn* wind-wood (one yin) and *shào yīn* ministerial fire (one yang) contend and give rise to blockage in the throat. This reflects most, but certainly not all, clinical cases. When the classic states that the knotting of one yin and one yang is referred to as throat obstruction, this statement does not imply its inverse. That is, simply because the knotting of one yin and one yang causes throat obstruction does not mean that all cases of throat obstruction arise from the knotting of one yin and one yang.

Other statements from the *Inner Classic* such as the "knotting of two yang is called dispersion [disorder], the knotting of three yang is called diaphragm [disorder], and the knotting of three yin is called water [swelling]" all should be viewed in a similar way.[4]

PHYSICIAN A   How is it that throat disorders appear as part of deficiency-cold patterns?

DR. YU   One cause is related to constitutional considerations and the other is a reference to the misguided use of Western and Chinese medicinal substances. The constitutional

....

3. This consists of Pinelliae Rhizoma praeparatum *(zhì bàn xià)*, Cinnamomi Ramulus *(guì zhī)*, and Glycyrrhizae Radix *(gān cǎo)*.

4. *Translators' note:* At present, most take the two yang to refer to the two *yáng míng* channels (Stomach and Large Intestine). When these are both knotted up there is dryness that can lead to dispersion, or unquenchable thirst. The knotting of the three yang is thought to be related to the *tài yáng* channels (Small Intestine, Bladder). Knotting of these means that the lower orifices do not eliminate, while the upper orifices cannot receive. The result is a blockage of the two lower orifices (for urine and stool) with resultant counterflow of Stomach and Lung qi upward that affects the diaphragm, leading to reduced intake of food and drink. This is referred to as diaphragm disorder. Three yin is thought to refer to the *tài yīn* (Lung and Spleen) channels. Knotting of these prevents the Spleen from properly distributing the fluids derived from food and drink, while the Lung does not direct fluids downward to be excreted. This results in water retention and water swelling.

considerations refer to the fact that after attack from an external pathogen, the expression of the disorder and its subsequent development and transformations depend on the nature of the patient's constitution. This is not peculiar to throat disorders; all disorders are this way. The *Golden Mirror of the Medical Tradition (Yī zōng jīn jiàn)* expresses the clinically-derived thinking used by myself and my predecessors when it states that:

> Disorders of the six channels fall under the purview of cold damage, how is it then that, though the qi is the same, the disease differs [qi here refers to the six qi: dampness, cold, heat, wind, summerheat, and dryness]? Multiple outcomes stem from the differences in each body's frame and organs. Understanding the meaning of mutual domination of water and fire, what difficulty is there in [grasping] the concept of cold and heat transformations?

This passage, taken from the section entitled "Complete details of cold damage transmission [where] heat transforms from yang and cold transforms from yin," is profound and enlightening and can lead to many insights in the clinic.

The misguided use of Western and Chinese medicinal substances can be seen in cases of throat disorders where the original cause is fire. Because of the unrestrained use of cold and cool herbs and drugs and the resultant lurking heat and fire (cold congeals and traps pathogenic heat deep in the body), the cold and heat together overcome the qi that generates the body's yang. Over time, yang deficiency and congealed cold give rise to a deficiency-cold pattern.

It is worth noting that many doctors nowadays, upon seeing throat disorders, fail to differentiate the hot and cold, excess and deficient, and chronic or temporary nature of the pattern. These practitioners have a tendency to indiscriminately prescribe bitter, cold, heat-clearing herbs like Forsythiae Fructus *(lián qiào)*, Lonicerae Flos *(jīn yín huā)*, Belamcandae Rhizoma *(shè gān)*, Sophorae tonkinensis Radix *(shān dòu gēn)*, Isatidis Folium *(dà qīng yè)*, and Isatidis/Baphicacanthis Radix *(bǎn lán gēn)*.

5.2 Throat and oral cavity

Six years of canker sores

Treating illness is easy, nourishing the Heart is difficult

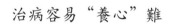

治病容易 "養心" 難

■ CASE HISTORY

Patient: *35-year-old woman*

Six years previously the patient developed canker sores in her mouth for the first time. The first sores appeared on the inside of her lower lip and on the roof of her mouth. At the time she took the patent medicine Coptis Pill to Clear the Upper *(huáng lián shàng qīng wán)*, which helped resolve the problem.

However, after this she began having more outbreaks. These occurred during her menses or whenever she was run-down, hadn't had enough sleep, or ate spicy food. On these occasions she took an assortment of Chinese and Western medicines until the sores would finally resolve, which usually took about ten days.

Most commonly, the locations of the outbreaks were the inside of her lips, the palate, or on the inside of her left cheek. Over the past three years the canker sores erupted more and more frequently until it got to the point that as one sore was healing, at least one other would begin to appear. It seemed she always had a sore somewhere in her mouth.

She was diagnosed as having recurrent oral ulcers by biomedical doctors, who told her to eat more fruit and fresh vegetables and to take a multivitamin supplement. She was also told to use antibiotics and steroids as well as apply Borneol and Borax Powder *(bīng péng sǎn)* when the sores became severe. The patient had previously taken over a hundred doses of Augmented Rambling Powder *(jiā wèi xiāo yáo sǎn)*, Anemarrhena, Phellodendron, and Rehmannia Pill *(zhī bǎi dì huáng wán)*, Five-Ingredient Drink to Eliminate Toxin *(wǔ wèi xiāo dú yǐn)*, and Emperor of Heaven's Special Pill to Tonify the Heart *(tiān wáng bǔ xīn dān)*, which at times seemed to help, but never markedly so. Nothing she tried ever truly controlled the recurrence of her symptoms.

Intake Examination
September 22, 1987

The patient suffered from fatigue and her complexion was wan. She had an ulcer on her inner lower lip, one on her palate, and one on the inside of her left cheek. The sores were round, about the size of a soybean, yellow, and concave in the middle and red around the edges. She said that the sores were painful and her sleep was restless. She also reported having a dry throat, yellow urine, and stools that tended to be dry. Her tongue was red with scant moisture and a greasy, yellow coating. Her pulse was weak and slightly rapid.

Differential Diagnosis and Discussion of Treatment

PHYSICIAN A   Dr. Yu, you often place great value in using a particular formula for a specific disease, and a specific formula for a specific pattern. You also, assuming that the differentiation is accurate and the treatment method proper, promote trying to choose and verify the efficacy of particular formulas that aim to treat a particular illness and that will bring rapid results. You also advance the notion that once there is confidence in the efficacy of such an approach, it should be publicized to the medical field. Can a specialized formula be found that is appropriate for the type of condition we are looking at here?

DR. YU   Recurrent stomatitis, commonly referred to as canker sores, presents in the context of many different patterns. For example, Spleen yin deficiency with flaring ascent of deficiency fire and lingering damp-heat; excess heat in the Triple Burner with concurrent damp-heat; Liver-Spleen disharmony with heat due to constraint; deficiency cold; or yin deficiency with concurrent damp-heat. Based on the patient's symptoms, this case was initially diagnosed as yin deficiency with damp-heat. For this pattern a modified Sweet Dew Drink *(gān lù yǐn)* is *the* specific formula.

PHYSICIAN A Are you saying that Sweet Dew Drink *(gān lù yǐn)* is the specific formula for mouth sores due to yin deficiency with damp-heat?

DR. YU Yes, that's what I am saying. But this isn't to say that mouth sores are the only disorder that this formula treats. Sweet Dew Drink *(gān lù yǐn)* is discussed in the *Medical Formulas Collected and Analyzed (Yī fāng jí jiě)*, where it says that it "treats damp-heat in the Stomach, [with] mouth odor and sores in the throat, [where the] roots of the teeth are exposed and there is spitting of blood due to bleeding from the teeth." Hence, it is clear that the scope of application of this formula goes beyond simply treating mouth sores.

A friend of mine, the eminent doctor from Leshan, Chen Si-Yi, once treated a patient with a stubborn case of cough and wheezing. The patient's tongue was red and completely covered with a thick and greasy, yellow coating. Dr. Chen repeatedly gave the patient herbs to clear heat and calm wheezing but they weren't effective, and the thick, greasy, yellow tongue coating didn't diminish. The patient then went to see an old doctor in his seventies who prescribed three packets of Sweet Dew Drink *(gān lù yǐn)*. The patient's coughing and wheezing greatly subsided and the thick, greasy, yellow tongue coating was reduced by more than half. The doctor continued with a combination of Sweet Dew Drink *(gān lù yǐn)* and Six Gentlemen Decoction to Tonify Metal and Water *(jīn shuǐ liù jūn jiān)* to finish the treatment. Dr. Chen heard about this, stomped his foot and sighed, "I have deep regret that my assessment lacked insight. From now on I will view this formula with greater respect."

Clinical practice has shown that this formula can be used for many conditions that are due to yin deficiency either with concurrent damp-heat or complicated by damp-heat. Sometimes it is possible to get unexpectedly remarkable results.

Treatment and Outcome

FIRST VISIT: We concluded that the patient had a pattern of yin depletion of the Stomach and Kidney with accumulation and steaming of damp-heat.

Treatment: Enrich and nourish the Stomach and Kidney, clear and transform damp-heat.

The patient was given six packets of the following modification of Sweet Dew Drink *(gān lù yǐn)*:

Asparagi Radix *(tiān mén dōng)*	12g
Ophiopogonis Radix *(mài mén dōng)*	12g
Rehmanniae Radix *(shēng dì huáng)*	10g
Rehmanniae Radix praeparata *(shú dì huáng)*	10g
Scutellariae Radix *(huáng qín)*	10g
Aurantii Fructus *(zhǐ ké)*	10g
Dendrobii Herba *(shí hú)*	10g
Artemisiae scopariae Herba *(yīn chén)*	10g
Glycyrrhizae Radix *(gān cǎo)*	5g
Polygoni cuspidati Rhizoma *(hǔ zhàng)*	15g
Taraxaci Herba *(pú gōng yīng)*	15g
Eriobotryae Folium *(pí pá yè)*	25g

The patient was advised to avoid acrid and spicy foods.

SECOND VISIT: Traces of the sores were still evident, but by and large, the ulcers had healed, and the burning sensation around them had markedly diminished. The patient's tongue was slightly red with a thin and yellow coating. Her pulse was still weak.

THIRD VISIT: There were no longer any visible remnants of the sores, the patient was in good spirits, and her complexion was glowing. She reported that both her appetite and sleep were excellent.

In order to consolidate the treatment, a modified Ginseng, Poria, and White Atractylodes Powder *(shēn líng bái zhú sǎn)* was prescribed:

Pseudostellariae Radix *(tài zǐ shēn)*	60g
Glehniae Radix *(běi shā shēn)*	60g
Polygonati odorati Rhizoma *(yù zhú)*	60g
Atractylodis macrocephalae Rhizoma *(bái zhú)*	60g
Poria *(fú líng)*	60g
Glycyrrhizae Radix *(gān cǎo)*	60g
Dioscoreae Rhizoma *(shān yào)*	60g
Cistanches Herba *(ròu cōng róng)*	60g
Cassiae Semen *(jué míng zǐ)*	60g
Nelumbinis Semen *(lián zǐ)*	30g
Platycodi Radix *(jié gěng)*	30g
Coicis Semen *(yì yǐ rén)*	30g
Lablab Semen album *(bái biǎn dòu)*	30g
Dendrobii Herba *(shí hú)*	30g
Trichosanthis Radix *(tiān huā fěn)*	30g
Polygoni cuspidati Rhizoma *(hǔ zhàng)*	30g
Amomi Fructus *(shā rén)*	15g
charred Phellodendri Cortex *(jiāo huáng bǎi)*	15g
Gigeriae galli Endothelium corneum *(jī nèi jīn)*	15g

Instructions: Roast the herbs under a low heat until crisp, grind them to a fine powder, and combine with honey to make pills, each pill weighing about 10g. One pill was to be taken three times each day for 50 days.

RESULT: Two years after she first saw me, the patient returned to the hospital to be treated for an unrelated condition. She told us that she had not had a single recurrence of mouth sores since the time of her treatment.

Disease	Primary symptoms	Differential diagnosis	Treatment method	Formula
Canker sores	Recurrent canker sores, red tongue with yellow, greasy coating	Stomach and Kidney yin depletion, accumulation and steaming of damp-heat	Enrich and nourish the Stomach and Kidney, clear and transform warm-heat	Sweet Dew Drink *(gān lù yǐn)*

REFLECTIONS AND CLARIFICATIONS

PHYSICIAN A Sweet Dew Drink *(gān lù yǐn)* is a good choice for treating recurrent canker sores if they are due to yin deficiency with concurrent damp-heat. In this patient's case her tongue coating was yellow and greasy. This signaled that the damp-heat was particularly severe. The formula you prescribed, Sweet Dew Drink *(gān lù yǐn)*, contains Asparagi Radix *(tiān mén dōng)* and Ophiopogonis Radix *(mài mén dōng)* along with both Rehmanniae Radix *(shēng dì huáng)* and Rehmanniae Radix praeparata *(shú dì huáng)*, which are quite cloying. How was it that these herbs didn't hinder the elimination of dampness, and that her tongue coating improved?

DR. YU In a pattern of yin deficiency with concurrent damp-heat it is advisable to simultaneously nourish yin and fluids and clear and facilitate the removal of damp-heat. However, if we choose not to use already established formulas that have been tested throughout the ages and found to be effective and reliable, and instead rashly put together our own creation or randomly choose some yin-enriching herbs along with some heat-clearing and dampness-resolving ones, we will end up with the situation of "having herbs but no formula." This will make it very difficult to get the desired results.

Sweet Dew Drink *(gān lù yǐn)*, as it's constructed in the *Formulary of the Pharmacy Service for Benefitting the People in the Taiping Era (Tài píng huì mín hé jì jú fang)*, is very effective in treating yin-deficiency, damp-heat canker sores, and it is certainly more effective than other similar formulas. Within the formula, Asparagi Radix *(tiān mén dōng)*, Ophiopogonis Radix *(mài mén dōng)*, Rehmanniae Radix *(shēng dì huáng)*, Rehmanniae Radix praeparata *(shú dì huáng)*, Dendrobii Herba *(shí hú)*, and Glycyrrhizae Radix *(gān cǎo)* are used together to enrich and nourish Stomach and Kidney yin. Scutellariae Radix *(huáng qín)* and Artemisiae scopariae Herba *(yīn chén)* are used to clear heat and resolve dampness, while Aurantii Fructus *(zhǐ ké)* diffuses and benefits the qi dynamic. But what makes the formula extraordinary is the use of a large dosage of Eriobotryae Folium *(pí pá yè)* to disseminate Lung qi and cause it to descend (the Lung governs qi, and qi transformation leads to the transformation of damp-heat).

This formula has been used by many physicians throughout history because of its ability to nourish yin/fluids without trapping damp-heat, and to clear heat and resolve dampness without damaging the yin and fluids. The late Ming-dynasty physician Wang Ken-Tang, in his book *Essential Manual of the Divine Orchid (Líng lán yào lǎn)*, recorded a case study involving the use of this formula:

> Mr. Yan Wen-Jing from Changshu was more than 70-years old but was still sexually active. He consumed countless warm tonics, as well as ginseng cooked in porridge and thick soups made with Cistanches Herba *(ròu cōng róng)*. This caused Stomach heat, and he developed numerous eroding ulcers in his mouth, loose teeth, and his breath was so foul it was almost impossible to get near him. He repeatedly took cold and cool Stomach-clearing medicines, but these were ineffective. He had a desire to add ginger and cinnamon as paradoxical assistants in the formulas he was taking. He asked my opinion. I said, "If ginger and cinnamon are used there will be severe consequences." [I recommended] a modified Sweet Dew Drink *(gān lù yǐn)* as the primary formula. After eight packets the symptoms were gone.

This is similar to the experience of the mid-Qing-dynasty physician Chen Xiu-Yuan, who, despite revering the classics and the ancients, admitted that this post-classical-era formula was excellent at both enriching yin and resolving dampness. In his opinion, the use of Ophiopogonis Radix *(mài mén dōng)* and Asparagi Radix *(tiān mén dōng)* in this formula was similar to the use of Asini Corii Colla *(ē jiāo)* in the formula Polyporus Decoction *(zhū líng tāng)* from the *Discussion of Cold Damage (Sháng hán lùn)* for nourishing yin, while Scutellariae Radix *(huáng qín)*, Artemisiae scopariae Herba *(yīn chén)* and Aurantii Fructus *(zhǐ ké)* in Sweet Dew Drink *(gān lù yǐn)* are used in a way comparable to how Talcum *(huá shí)* and Alismatis Rhizoma *(zé xiè)* are used in Polyporus Decoction *(zhū líng tāng)* to promote the resolution of dampness and eliminate filth.

One needn't worry about using Sweet Dew Drink *(gān lù yǐn)* to treat any yin-deficiency pattern with concurrent damp-heat, regardless of how yellow and greasy the patient's tongue coating may be.

PHYSICIAN B Besides using Sweet Dew Drink *(gān lù yǐn)* to treat canker sores, you are also keen on using a formula devised by the late-Qing physician Zheng Qin-An, Special Pill to Seal the Marrow *(fēng suǐ dān)*, for this condition. This formula, which consists of Amomi Fructus *(shā rén)*, Phellodendri Cortex *(huáng bǎi)*, and Glycyrrhizae Radix *(gān cǎo)*, was originally used to treat seminal loss and night sweats due to exuberant ministerial fire. How can this formula also be effective in treating mouth sores?

DR. YU Some cases of recurrent canker sores are due to three patterns in combination: Spleen yin deficiency, flaring ascent of deficiency fire, and lingering damp-heat. These factors influence and aggravate each other.

Early in my career I treated this pattern with a modified combination of Shen-Rou's Decoction to Nourish the True *(Shèn-Róu yáng zhēn tāng)*[5] and Ginseng, Poria, and White Atractylodes Powder *(shēn líng bái zhú sǎn)*. However, the effects weren't as good as I would have liked. It wasn't until I learned from the experience of the famous 20th-century physician Pu Fu-Zhou and used a modified version of Special Pill to Seal the Marrow *(fēng suǐ dān)* that my results improved.

Traditionally, Special Pill to Seal the Marrow *(fēng suǐ dān)* was primarily used to treat a pattern of exuberant ministerial fire with instability of Kidney essence. It was only master Pu who had the insight to see this as a formula that tonifies earth and subdues fire, and that it could be used to treat recurrent canker sores owing to deficient earth with flaring ascent of floating fire. A brilliant idea, but used by itself, the formula's ability to tonify Spleen yin and resolve dampness is insufficient. Hence, it's necessary to add herbs to achieve that goal.

I usually use 10g each of Glycyrrhizae Radix *(gān cǎo)*, Amomi Fructus *(shā rén)*, and charred Phellodendri Cortex *(jiāo huáng bǎi)*, then add 10g of Dendrobii Herba

5. This comes from the mid-17th century work *Five Texts by [Hu] Shen-Rou (Shèn-Róu wǔ shū)* and consists of Ginseng Radix *(rén shēn)*, Glycyrrhizae Radix *(gān cǎo)*, Poria *(fú líng)*, Atractylodis macrocephalae Rhizoma *(bái zhú)*, Astragali Radix *(huáng qí)*, Dioscoreae Rhizoma *(shān yào)*, Nelumbinis Semen *(lián zǐ)*, Schisandrae Fructus *(wǔ wèi zǐ)*, and Ophiopogonis Radix *(mài mén dōng)*.

(shí hú) to nourish Spleen yin, and 12g of Paeoniae Radix alba *(bái sháo)* to not only restrain the Liver to prevent it from insulting the Spleen, but also, when combined with Glycyrrhizae Radix *(gān căo)*, it forms Peony and Licorice Decoction *(sháo yào gān căo tāng)*. This combination of sour and sweet herbs generates and nourishes yin. According to the system of the Ten Heavenly Stems, 甲 *jiă* (associated with wood, as is the sour flavor) and 乙 *jǐ* (associated with earth, as is the sweet flavor) together transform earth and can tonify the Spleen. Hence, this is an excellent formula for treating Spleen yin. The further addition of 10g of Phragmitis Rhizoma *(lú gēn)* and 6g of Succinum *(hŭ pò)* (taken as powder) helps to guide the accumulated damp-heat downwards.

I'd like to share some information about this formula garnered from my experience: the Glycyrrhizae Radix *(gān căo)* in the formula must be unprocessed. Not only does unprocessed Glycyrrhizae Radix *(gān căo)* tonify the Spleen and subdue fire, it also clears heat and resolves toxicity. Initially the dosage of Glycyrrhizae Radix *(gān căo)* should be larger than normal, up to 10g. With this dosage the effects will be much faster, but this dosage should not be continued long-term out of concern that the patient will experience fullness and swelling. Once there are signs that the formula is working, the Glycyrrhizae Radix *(gān căo)*, Amomi Fructus *(shā rén)*, and charred Phellodendri Cortex *(jiāo huáng băi)* can each be reduced to 6g to continue with a gentler strategy. Another option for use of this formula is to roast all the herbs, grind them into a fine powder and take 3g, three times a day. When the mouth sores begin to disappear, don't immediately discontinue the herbs. It is beneficial to continue with them for approximately two weeks after symptoms have dissipated in order to consolidate the effect.

My experience has taught me that although there are numerous patterns that result in recurrent canker sores, yin deficiency with damp-heat is far and away the most common underlying pattern. If you can make good use of these two formulas—Sweet Dew Drink *(gān lù yĭn)* and Special Pill to Seal the Marrow *(fēng suĭ dān)*—to treat canker sores, you will have figured out most of what you need to know.

PHYSICIAN B How about those cases that don't present as yin deficiency with damp-heat? How do you treat them?

DR. YU If the sores are due to Triple Burner excess heat with concurrent damp-heat, then it's best to drain fire and resolve toxicity, clear heat, and resolve dampness. Coptis Decoction to Resolve Toxicity *(huáng lián jiě dú tāng)* together with a modified version of Five-Ingredient Drink to Eliminate Toxin *(wŭ wèi xiāo dú yĭn)* is useful. If the cause is Liver and Spleen disharmony with accompanying damp-heat due to constraint, then dredging the Liver, supporting the Spleen, opening areas of constraint, and discharging fire is the best method. For this, consider a modified Augmented Rambling Powder *(jiā wèi xiāo yáo săn)*.

These patterns are not difficult to differentiate or treat. One thing worth paying attention to, however, is the occasional case of deficiency-cold mouth sores. This type has its own unique characteristics, including the sores themselves and the area around the sores tend to be pale or grayish white, and cold medicinal substances aggravate the patient's symptoms.

If, in addition to these symptoms, the patient also presents with mental lassitude and fatigue, spontaneous sweating, reluctance to speak, poor appetite and loose stools, this indicates Spleen deficiency with sinking qi and fire leaving its proper location and gushing upward. Treatment should be directed at tonifying the Spleen, raising sunken qi, and draining yin fire. Tonify the Middle to Augment the Qi Decoction (bǔ zhōng yì qì tāng) together with Special Pill to Seal the Marrow (fēng suǐ dān), limiting charred Phellodendri Cortex (jiao huáng bǎi) to 3g, can be prescribed.

If a patient with deficiency-cold mouth sores also has a cold body and limbs, abdominal pain and loose stools, this indicates Spleen and Kidney yang deficiency with internal abundance of yin/cold that is pushing the yang to float upward. Treatment should be aimed at tonifying the Spleen and Kidney, breaking up yin, and returning yang to its source. In mild cases of this pattern, use Cinnamon and Prepared Aconite Accessory Root Decoction to Regulate the Middle (guì fù lǐ zhōng tang). For more severe cases, use Unblock the Pulse Decoction for Frigid Extremities (tōng mài sì nì tāng).

Some physicians are afraid of using warm or hot herbs to treat canker sores. As a matter of fact, warm and hot herbs can be used not only for canker sores, but also for mouth erosions (口糜 kǒu mǐ)—similar to some infectious diseases of the oral mucosa in biomedicine, which are characterized by vesicular erythematous erosions.

This has already been documented in the *Essential Manual of the Divine Orchid (Líng lán yào lǎn)* where it notes:

> [My] nephew came down with a very severe case of mouth erosions, and the heat was so severe that he only desired to drink cold [fluids]. I gave him 2g each of Ginseng Radix (rén shēn), Atractylodis macrocephalae Rhizoma (bái zhú), Zingiberis Rhizoma (gān jiāng), with 1g each of Poria (fú líng) and Glycyrrhizae Radix (gān cǎo), which was decocted and taken cold. After a few doses he recovered. It is impossible to talk to physicians who are stuck in their ways of prescribing about this type of treatment.

This passage goes on to say:

> For those who have taken cool medicinal substances and [their symptoms have] not resolved, this is due to overconsumption of alcohol and food, or overwork with insomnia. The tongue is glossy and peeled. Or it may be that worry and pensiveness have damaged the middle qi and deficiency fire has spilled upward unchecked. Use Regulate the Middle Decoction (lǐ zhōng tāng) to treat. If severe, add Aconiti Radix lateralis praeparata (zhì fù zǐ) and Cinnamomi Cortex (ròu guì) held in the mouth.

Because of the 'yin fire' characteristic of this type of canker sore or mouth erosion, its nature is cold and so don't avoid warm or hot medicinal substances. In fact, it's imperative to use them to warm the channels and disperse cold.

PHYSICIAN B   In Western biomedicine canker sores are thought to be the result of vitamin deficiencies. But even with vitamin supplementation it is difficult to see results. With Chinese medicine the short-term results are better, but to really get to the root and keep recurrence under control is still a challenge. Is this your experience Dr. Yu?

DR. YU   The way I see it, rather than say "vitamin deficiency" it would be better to say that the body's ability to absorb nutrients has diminished. In recent years biomedicine's understanding of this illness has deepened. It is now considered that there is some relationship between this condition and defects of cellular immunity and t-lymphocyte dysfunction. Consequently, even biomedicine is often adopting the TCM method of "supporting the normal qi and expelling the pathogen."

This raises the issue of Chinese medicine's ability to treat stubborn cases and thoroughly prevent recurrences. Early on in my studies I felt that there was a strong relationship between this illness and constitutional factors. However, my clinical experience has taught me that treating disease is relatively easy and improving someone's constitution is not that difficult. What's difficult is thoroughly changing the pathological constitution: making qi perform its job of warming, and blood to do its job of moistening, conserving yin, and keeping yang concealed. This involves the primary issue of nourishing both the body and the Heart, along with improving the natural and social environments in which we live. To use a couple of fashionable phrases, this "systems engineering" issue needs some "comprehensive management." By no means can this problem be completely solved by special medicines alone.

5.3 Nasal congestion

Three years of nasal congestion and diminished sense of smell

Obtaining quick results reinforces patient confidence

取其述效增強患者信心

■ **CASE HISTORY**

Patient: *Mr. Li, 36-year-old male*

Three years ago the patient had a recurring cold that lasted two months. After the cold abated, nasal congestion remained. Mr. Li did not pay much attention to it and treated the condition with nasal drops (some of which were ephedrine-based). Initially, these temporarily opened his nasal passages, but after a time the relief provided by these remedies gradually decreased. In addition, the patient's sense of smell began to diminish.

Over the last two years the patient has taken the patent medicine Rhinitis Pills *(bí yán piàn)*[6] over an extended period, while off and on taking decoctions of formulas such as Xanthium Powder *(cāng ěr zǐ sǎn)*, Special Pill to Warm the Lung and Stop Flow *(wēn fèi zhǐ liú dān)*,[7] and Unblock the Orifices and Invigorate the Blood Decoction *(tōng qiào huó*

....

6. *Translators' note:* There are many patent medicines by this name. One common one contains Bupleuri Radix *(chái hú)*, Menthae haplocalycis Herba *(bò hé)*, Chrysanthemi Flos *(jú huā)*, Viticis Fructus *(màn jīng zǐ)*, Saposhnikoviae Radix *(fáng fēng)*, Schizonepetae Spica *(jīng jiè suì)*, Scutellariae Radix *(huáng qín)*, Platycodi Radix *(jié gěng)*, Chuanxiong Rhizoma *(chuān xiōng)*, Angelicae dahuricae Radix *(bái zhǐ)*, Aurantii Fructus *(zhǐ ké)*, Bubali Cornu *(shuǐ niú jiǎo)*, Asari Radix et Rhizoma *(xì xīn)*, Gentianae Radix *(lóng dǎn cǎo)*, and Magnoliae Flos *(xīn yí)*.

7. This is a formula by the Qing-dynasty physician Chen Shi-Duo. It includes Ginseng Radix

xuè tāng). Each time Mr. Li would begin a formula there would seem to be some effect, but over time there was no noticeable improvement. He almost lost hope for a successful treatment.

INTAKE EXAMINATION
NOVEMBER 25, 1985

The patient reported that on days when the temperature was mild his nasal congestion was less severe or would be variable (with nighttime congestion alternating between the left and right nostrils depending on which side he was lying on). When the weather was colder, however, the congestion was more severe and continuous. He had frequent colds which were accompanied by nasal mucus that was either copious and white or thick and pale yellow. His sense of smell was not acute and he had difficulty distinguishing between fragrant and unpleasant scents. His food intake was acceptable and his stools and urine were normal. His pulse and tongue also had no obvious abnormalities. Examination of his nasal cavity revealed swelling and distention in the mucous membranes, a swollen pair of lower turbinates, and some pale yellow, sticky nasal mucus. The biomedical diagnosis was chronic, simple rhinitis.

DIFFERENTIATION OF PATTERNS AND DISCUSSION OF TREATMENT

PHYSICIAN A   Chronic, simple rhinitis equates to nasal blockage (鼻窒 *bí zhì*) in Chinese medical terminology. Although this disorder is not a serious one, it nonetheless lingers and is difficult to treat. Moreover, it can easily develop into hypertrophic or atrophic rhinitis, both of which are even more intractable. A great many chronic rhinitis patients who simply take herbs internally do not achieve results, especially ones that last; this leaves them very distressed.

DR. YU   It is well known that nasal blockage's fundamental pathodynamic has two aspects. The first is a deficient constitution where the Spleen, Lung, and Kidney are deficient, so the clear yang does not rise into the upper body. The second aspect is excess in the exterior; notably, a congealed, stagnant, turbid pathogen in the orifices of the nose. Regardless of which formula is chosen to treat this condition, it is necessary to use as guiding herbs those that open the orifices and allow free flow through blocked areas. In this way, the formula will be guided to the site of the disorder where it can be effective. Therefore, the appropriate use of these guiding herbs to open the orifices and allow free flow through areas of blockage is truly crucial.

The most well-known herb for unblocking nasal congestion is Magnoliae Flos *(xīn yí)*. But when it is decocted, many of this herb's effective aspects are destroyed, and if put into pills, its effective aspects do not completely express themselves. Therefore, it is only when powdered that most of the effective aspects of this herb are preserved and can be utilized.

I conducted an experiment as follows. We roasted one kilogram of Magnoliae Flos *(xīn yí)* over a low flame until it was crisp and then ground it to a fine powder. We

....
(rén shēn), Schizonepetae Herba *(jīng jiè),* Platycodi Radix *(jié gěng),* Chebulae Fructus *(hē zǐ),* Pogostemonis/Agastaches Herba *(huò xiāng),* Asari Radix et Rhizoma *(xì xīn),* and Glycyrrhizae Radix *(gān cǎo).*

selected ten patients with chronic rhinitis and had them take 6g of the powder with warm water three times per day. We asked them to cease all other treatment (including nasal drops). Upon follow-up we learned that after three days, all ten patients had seen improvement. The most rapid change was observed after just one dose. The patients felt that their nasal cavities were unobstructed. Not long after, however, the congestion returned. This experiment demonstrated that herbs that open the orifices and open congested areas have difficulty treating the root of the disorder.

So, how do we treat the root of nasal blockage?

There is a chapter entitled "Discussion of Blockage of the Nine Orifices from Deficiency of the Spleen and Stomach" in Li Dong Yuan's *Discussion of Spleen and Stomach Damage (Pí wèi lùn)* in which he quotes Chapter 19 of the *Basic Questions (Sū wèn)*, that when the Spleen is "inadequate, it leads to blockage of a person's nine orifices." He also refers to Chapter 28 of the *Basic Questions (Sū wèn)*, which states that lack of free passage through the nine orifices is generated in the Intestines and Stomach. Li Dong-Yuan expounds on this in his *Discussion of the Spleen and Stomach (Pí wèi lùn)* by stating "[the] Spleen and Stomach are overwhelmed by yin fire, the grain qi is blocked and flows downward. Thus, the clear qi cannot ascend [and the] nine orifices lose free flow."

The nose is one of the nine orifices and in the investigation into the root of long-term nasal congestion and diminished sense of smell it is natural to first suspect deficient weakness of the Spleen and Stomach, as this leads to failure of the clear yang to ascend and the turbid yin to descend.

Treatment and Outcome

Chinese medicine diagnosis: Nasal blockage

Magnoliae Flos *(xīn yí)* 54g

Instructions: Roast over a low flame until crisp and then grind to a fine powder. Take three times per day, 6g each time, washed down with warm water. Continue for three days and cease all other medications.

Second visit: December 5. After taking the herbs twice the patient felt that his congestion was somewhat improved. After taking all of the herbs, Mr. Li's congestion was just about gone, and his sense of smell had returned. Three days after he stopped taking the herbs, however, his stuffiness returned, and he once again found it difficult to distinguish smells.

Tonify the Middle to Augment the Qi Decoction *(bǔ zhōng yì qì tāng)* combined with Jade Windscreen Powder *(yù píng fēng sǎn)* and Reed Decoction *(wěi jīng tāng)* with additions of Aucklandiae Radix *(mù xiāng)* and Magnoliae Flos *(xīn yí)* were prescribed:

Astragali Radix *(huáng qí)* 30g
Codonopsis Radix *(dǎng shēn)* 15g
Atractylodis macrocephalae Rhizoma *(bái zhú)* 12g
Glycyrrhizae Radix praeparata *(zhì gān cǎo)* 5g
Cimicifugae Rhizoma *(shēng má)* 6g
Bupleuri Radix *(chái hú)* 6g
Citri reticulatae Pericarpium *(chén pí)* 10g
Aucklandiae Radix *(mù xiāng)* 30g

> Saposhnikoviae Radix *(fáng fēng)* 10g
> Magnoliae Flos *(xīn yí)*
>   [roasted, powdered and taken with the strained decoction]........... 10g
> Persicae Semen *(táo rén)*... 10g
> Benincasae Semen *(dōng guā zǐ)*................................... 30g
> Coicis Semen *(yì yǐ rén)*... 30g
> Phragmitis Rhizoma *(lú gēn)*[8] 30g
> Jujubae Fructus *(dà zǎo)* 12g
> Zingiberis Rhizoma recens *(shēng jiāng)*......................... 6g

Instructions: Take 20 packets continuously, even in the event of catching a cold.

THIRD VISIT: March 12, 1986

After taking six packets of the above formula the patient's nasal passages gradually cleared; after 20 packets the passages were completely cleared, and his sense of smell was comparatively intact. This period was at the height of winter and still Mr. Li did not catch any colds. Lately, with the weather fluctuating between warm and cold spells, occasionally the patient has experienced some minor nasal stuffiness. The following was prescribed:

> Astragali Radix *(huáng qí)*................................... 100g
> Angelicae sinensis Radix *(dāng guī)*........................... 50g
> Salviae miltiorrhizae Radix *(dān shēn)*........................ 50g
> Cuscutae Semen *(tù sī zǐ)*................................... 100g
> Morindae officinalis Radix *(bā jǐ tiān)*........................ 100g
> Magnoliae Flos *(xīn yí)*...................................... 50g
> Angelicae dahuricae Radix *(bái zhǐ)*[9] 20g

Instructions: Take 10g of powder with warm water three times per day. Do not take these herbs while having a cold. Roast all the substances until crisp and then grind to a powder. Store the powder in a closed, airtight container.

After he completed taking this formula the patient's nasal passages became entirely cleared and his olfactory function returned to normal. Examination by the Ear, Nose, and Throat Department revealed no abnormalities in his nasal cavities. The patient had had no recurrences on a follow-up visit one year later.

Disease	Primary symptoms	Differential diagnosis	Treatment method	Formula
Nasal blockage	Stuffy nose and diminished sense of smell	Exhaustion and deficiency in the Lung and Kidney; congealed, stagnant, turbid pathogen in the nasal passages	Strengthen the Spleen, tonify the Lung, guide out turbidity and dispel stagnation	Tonify the Middle to Augment the Qi Decoction *(bǔ zhōng yì qì tāng)* combined with Jade Windscreen Powder *(yù píng fēng sǎn)* and Reed Decoction *(wěi jīng tāng)*

....

8. Dr. Yu believes that Phragmitis Rhizoma *(lú gēn)*, which is much easier to obtain, is just as good as Phragmititis Caulis *(wěi jīng)* here.

9. *Translators' note:* Dr. Yu originally used 5g of Moschus *(shè xiāng)*, which is very difficult to obtain, as well as being prohibitively expensive. This is a suggested substitute.

REFLECTIONS AND CLARIFICATIONS

PHYSICIAN B   Treating nasal blockage requires using herbs to unblock the orifices. The commonly used formulas to treat this condition, such as Rhinitis Pills *(bí yán piàn)* and Xanthium Powder *(cāng ěr zǐ sǎn)*, all use these herbs. In the present case, these formulas had already been tried without success, but in your first encounter with this patient you gave him the single herb Magnoliae Flos *(xīn yí)* to unblock the orifices. At that time, I thought that perhaps you were following in the tracks of a cart that had already been upended, and in fact that turned out to be the case.

DR. YU   The goal of prescribing the powdered Magnoliae Flos *(xīn yí)* in my first meeting with this patient was solely to temporarily clear his nasal passages. How could you expect it to eliminate the root of the disease?

   When I treat chronic rhinitis, I continue to be fond of initially using powder of Magnoliae Flos *(xīn yí)* because it gives quick results. This initial success increases the patient's confidence so that I can continue the treatment by attacking both the root and branch of the disorder. If one treats both root and branch in the first attempt and after several packets of herbs the patient's nose is still congested, some patients will be unwilling to persevere in taking herbs over the long term.

PHYSICIAN B   Upon seeing the patient the second time you simultaneously treated the branch and root, but I am puzzled at the choice of Tonify the Middle to Augment the Qi Decoction *(bǔ zhōng yì qì tāng)* because the patient did not display signs of middle burner deficiency weakness such as shortness of breath, weakness, reduced food intake, and laconic speech.

DR. YU   This is an excellent question that allows us to touch upon the clinical scope of Tonify the Middle to Augment the Qi Decoction *(bǔ zhōng yì qì tāng)*. Let me pose this question: Is Tonify the Middle to Augment the Qi Decoction *(bǔ zhōng yì qì tāng)* only appropriate for use in cases where a patient displays signs of systemic deficiency weakness such as shortness of breath, weakness, reduced food intake, and laconic speech? I can still remember Jiang Er-Xun successfully treating many disorders of the anterior and posterior yin with Tonify the Middle to Augment the Qi Decoction *(bǔ zhōng yì qì tāng)*, including long-term urinary incontinence, blood in the urine, intractable proteinuria, painful urinary dribbling disorder, irregular uterine bleeding, blood in the stool, constipation, diarrhea, and hemorrhoids. Among these cases, most completely lacked, or had very few, systemic symptoms such as shortness of breath, weakness, reduced food intake, and laconic speech.

   I previously did not have a complete understanding of this and asked Dr. Jiang for direction: "According to what criteria do you apply Tonify the Middle to Augment the Qi Decoction *(bǔ zhōng yì qì tāng)*?"

   He immediately replied, "Ponder what the *Divine Pivot (Líng shū)* says [in Chapter 28]: 'With insufficient middle qi, urination changes due to this and the Intestines suffer from noises due to this' and you can deduce the conclusion." At that time, I felt as though my eyes suddenly opened to a new world. As the *Divine Pivot (Líng shū)* says [in Chapter 1], "If one grasps the essence, a single explanation is sufficient. If one doesn't grasp the essence, then [any explanation] will be scattered and boundless." This is no lie!

PHYSICIAN A   In the present three-year case of nasal congestion with diminished sense of smell the patient took several courses of herbs to no effect. You then primarily employed Tonify the Middle to Augment the Qi Decoction *(bǔ zhōng yì qì tāng)* to tonify the Spleen and Lung. In the final stage you employed formulas that tonified qi, invigorated blood, warmed the Kidneys and opened the orifices to secure a long-term effect. In these herbs and formulas there is nothing striking or unusual, yet the treatment effect was precise and is worth further investigation and promotion.

At the second visit, you combined the base of Tonify the Middle to Augment the Qi Decoction *(bǔ zhōng yì qì tāng)* with Reed Decoction *(wěi jīng tāng)*, which is a formula that treats Lung abscess. This is difficult to understand.

DR. YU   The nose is the orifice of the Lung. Phlegm and turbidity from the Lung ascends to block the orifices of the nose, and over time, block the channels and vessels. Reed Decoction *(wěi jīng tāng)* contains Benincasae Semen *(dōng guā zǐ)* and Coicis Semen *(yì yǐ rén)* to dispel phlegm and direct turbidity downward, Phragmititis Caulis *(wěi jīng)* to clear and disseminate Lung qi, and Persicae Semen *(táo rén)* to invigorate blood and unblock the collaterals. Therefore, it can be co-opted for this condition. This formula, when combined with Tonify the Middle to Augment the Qi Decoction *(bǔ zhōng yì qì tāng)*, attacks and tonifies, simultaneously treating branch and root.

PHYSICIAN B   I am curious about your dosing of Aucklandiae Radix *(mù xiāng)*. This herb is commonly used to move qi and the usual dosage is below 10g; why, in this formula, is the dosage as high as 30g?

DR. YU   In small dosage, Aucklandiae Radix *(mù xiāng)* can be used to move qi; in large dosage, it can tonify qi. Of course, this is a controversial statement. In the case here, the large dosage of Aucklandiae Radix *(mù xiāng)* is first used for its tonifying function to increase the ability of Tonify the Middle to Augment the Qi Decoction *(bǔ zhōng yì qì tāng)* to tonify qi. Secondarily, it is included because of its ability to unblock the orifices (this herb is acrid, warm and fragrant; also, its nature is moistening and oily and its function of opening the orifices is long-lasting) and assist Reed Decoction *(wěi jīng tāng)* and Magnoliae Flos *(xīn yí)* to unblock the nasal passages.

It should be said that my use of a large dosage of Aucklandiae Radix *(mù xiāng)* to tonfy qi is not only supported by clinical experience, but also is documented in texts. For example, the *Comprehensive Outline of the Materia Medica (Běn cǎo gāng mù)* notes a discussion by the late-13th-century physician Wang Hao-Gu elucidating the function of Aucklandiae Radix *(mù xiāng)*:

> A materia medica states: governing weak qi and insufficient qi, [it] tonifies; unblocking clogged qi and guiding out all qi, [it] breaks; quieting the fetus and strengthening the Spleen and Stomach, [it] tonifies; dispelling periumbilical and hypochondriac firmness and masses, [it] breaks.

The *Comprehensive Outline of the Materia Medica (Běn cǎo gāng mù)* also references the discussion by the 16th-century author Wang Ji about the function of Aucklandiae Radix *(mù xiāng)*, stating:

> [When used] with herbs that tonify, it [assumes the role of] assistant, thus, tonification [occurs], [when used] with herbs that drain, it [assumes the role of] sovereign, thus, draining [occurs].

It was in my practice that I initially observed that adding a large dosage of Aucklandiae Radix *(mù xiāng)* to Tonify the Middle to Augment the Qi Decoction *(bǔ zhōng yì qì tāng)* brought results that were superior to the formula on its own. I hope that people will carry on this investigation.

5.4.1 Visual distortion

A case of visual distortion for six months

Unabashedly ask questions and remain open to insight

不恥下問而茅塞頓開

■ CASE HISTORY

Patient: *44-year-old man*

The patient reported obstruction and distortion in the visual field of his right eye for the last six months. His vision was distorted such that straight lines would appear curved, round objects would appear oval, and square objects would appear rhomboid. According to the ophthalmologic exam, his right eye appeared outwardly normal and his visual acuity was 0.5 (20/40). An examination of the fundus of the eye revealed evidence of diffuse retinal macular edema with round spots of oozing fluid. The biomedical diagnosis was central serous chorioretinopathy. He was treated with diazepam, Compounded Salvia tablets *(fù fāng dān shēn piàn)*,[10] vitamins, and a 10% potassium iodide solution for more than a month without any improvement.

He had also taken other Chinese herb formulas such as modifications of Augmented Preserve Vistas Formula *(zhù jǐng wán jiā jiǎn fāng)*, Augmented Rambling Powder *(jiā wèi xiāo yáo sǎn)*, Three-Seed Decoction *(sān rén tāng)*, and Restore the Spleen Decoction *(guī pí tāng)*. However, after more than 60 packets of these formulas, he reported no improvement in his symptoms. At that point, he began trying prepared medicines such as Lycium Fruit, Chrysanthemum, and Rehmannia Pill *(qǐ jú dì huáng wán)*, Dendrobium Pill for Night Vision *(shí hú yè guāng wán)*, and Clear Eye Obstructions Pill *(zhàng yǎn míng piàn)*.[11] Because none yielded any benefit, he lost confidence in treatment.

....

10. This consists of Salviae miltiorrhizae Radix *(dān shēn)*, Notoginseng Radix *(sān qī)*, and Borneolum *(bīng piàn)*.

11. This consists of Cistanches Herba *(ròu cōng róng)*, Lycii Fructus *(gǒu qǐ zǐ)*, Rehmanniae

Intake Examination
June 23, 1993

The vision in his right eye was blurry and distorted. He also reported fatigue, dizziness, poor appetite, and slightly loose stools. His tongue was pale red with a thin, white, greasy coating. His pulse was moderate and weak. The patient reported that he spent a significant amount of time bent over his desk and that he smoked cigarettes, drank alcohol, and preferred to drink cold beverages.

Differentiation of Patterns and Discussion of Treatment

PHYSICIAN A   In this case the outward appearance of the eye was normal, yet the patient experienced blurriness and visual distortion. Examination of the fundus revealed that there was diffuse retinal macular edema with round spots of oozing fluid. The biomedical diagnosis was central serous chorioretinopathy. Given that treatment with both Western and Chinese medicines for more than six months yielded no benefit, this disease was considered difficult to cure. How did you go about using a holistic conception of the body in your diagnosis and treatment planning?

DR. YU   The first step was to define the disease location. We are all familiar with the work of the late Chen Da-Fu, an esteemed contemporary physician from Sichuan who created a theory connecting the internal structure of the eye with the six channels. This theory was the result of Dr. Chen's graduate research into the classical literature of Chinese medicine combined with his extensive knowledge of fundoscopic exams and many years of deep study and extensive clinical practice. Dr. Chen created a system known as the 'inner structure of the eye in relation to the six channels.'[12] He unequivocally indicates that the retinal macular area, as defined in Western medicine, pertains to the Spleen in Chinese medicine.[13] Thus, pathological changes in the macula should be treated through the Spleen. This established the location of the disease.

The second step was to define the nature of the disease. Dr. Chen believed that "serous" diseases commonly occur in patients who

> experience overwork, overuse of vision, working long hours, and exhaustion because these lead to consumption of the true yin. Deficient Liver and Kidney yin then fails to properly nourish the eyes. Furthermore, when the Spleen no longer has a strong transportive function, the clear yang fails to rise and the turbid yin fails to descend. Water and dampness flood upward, accumulating and stagnating in the collaterals of the eyes and resulting in this disorder. Clinically, most patients with serous diseases have a deficiency pattern with accompanying excess.[14]

Radix praeparata *(shú dì huáng)*, Corni Fructus *(shān zhū yú)*, Buddlejae Flos *(mì měng huā)*, Chrysanthemi Flos *(jú huā)*, Cassiae Semen *(jué míng zǐ)*, Prinsepiae Nux *(ruì rén)*, Celosiae Semen *(qīng xiāng zǐ)*, Chuanxiong Rhizoma *(chuān xiōng)*, Astragali Radix *(huáng qí)*, and Polygonati Rhizoma *(huáng jīng)*.

12. Chen Da-Fu, *Methodology for Using the Six Channels in Ophthalmology (Yǎn kē liù jīng fǎ yào)*. Chengdu: Sichuan Science and Technology Press, 1978.

13. Luo Guo-Fen, *The Chinese Medicine Clinical Experience of Chen Da-Fu (Chén Dá-Fū zhōng yī kē lín chuáng jīng yàn)*. Chengdu: Sichuan Science and Technology Press, 1985.

14. Ibid.

In the case described above, evidence of flooding ascent of damp turbidity is seen in the diffuse retinal macular edema with round spots of oozing fluid. Considering the other presenting signs and symptoms, it is not difficult to see that this case belongs to a deficiency pattern with accompanying excess. This situation can be characterized as a lack of coordination between the ascending and descending functions of the Spleen and Stomach, and yin fire carrying that bears damp turbidity upward to flood the upper body.

In this way, by combining the microscopic and the macroscopic evaluations, I determined the disease location. By combining the local assessment with a holistic perspective, I was able to determine the nature of the disease. Simply assessing the patient from a holistic perspective causes one to miss the actual situation.

PHYSICIAN A   Are you saying that without the work of Dr. Chen you would have been groping your way in the dark?

DR. YU   Maybe not, because I would still be able to follow the traditional ophthalmological theories relating to reduced visual acuity and distorted vision. Modern Chinese medicine ophthalmology books frequently state that eye diseases, particularly those relating to the fundus of the eye, show no external signs as [the disease] is concealed within. The pathodynamic is one of essence and qi failing to nourish the eyes as a result of dysfunction within the organs, channels, and collaterals. This pathodynamic is generally seen in patients whose eyes have no apparent abnormality, but who nonetheless suffer from distorted vision and reduced visual acuity.

Going through this process of establishing the diagnosis through a combined analysis of all the information described above clearly led to a determination that the disease was centered in the Spleen. However, I was not at ease. Why? Because in traditional Chinese medicine, emphasis has always been placed on the role of the Liver and Kidney in eye diseases. It was very hard for me to cast off this fixed mode of thinking and not be influenced by it when considering an appropriate herbal formula for the patient.

Luckily, I had the theory of Dr. Chen to show me the correct path. It was like a light in a dark room. Who says that modern practitioners are unable to innovate as well as their predecessors?

TREATMENT AND OUTCOME

This case is one where the Spleen and Stomach have lost their ability to regulate ascent and descent, and yin fire bears damp turbidity upward to flood the upper body. It was appropriate to tonify the Spleen and raise the clear, harmonize the Stomach and direct the turbid downward, while draining and restraining yin fire.

I prescribed Li Dong-Yuan's Raise the Yang and Augment the Stomach Decoction (*shēng yáng yì wèi tāng*):

Astragali Radix *(huáng qí)*	30g
Codonopsis Radix *(dǎng shēn)*	15g
Atractylodis macrocephalae Rhizoma *(bái zhú)*	15g
Coptidis Rhizoma *(huáng lián)*	3g
standard Pinelliae Rhizoma praeparatum *(fǎ bàn xià)*	10g

Glycyrrhizae Radix *(gān cǎo)* 5g

Citri reticulatae Pericarpium *(chén pí)* 10g

Poria *(fú líng)* 15g

Alismatis Rhizoma *(zé xiè)* 30g

Saposhnikoviae Radix *(fáng fēng)* 10g

Notopterygii Rhizoma seu Radix *(qiāng huó)* 5g

Angelicae pubescentis Radix *(dú huó)* 5g

Bupleuri Radix *(chái hú)* 5g

Paeoniae Radix alba *(bái sháo)* 10g

Jujubae Fructus *(dà zǎo)* 10g

Zingiberis Rhizoma recens *(shēng jiāng)* 10g

I gave the patient six packets and advised him to temporarily suspend work activities, stop smoking, and to stop drinking alcohol and refrain from drinking cold liquids.

SECOND VISIT: The patient's dizziness had diminished, his appetite had improved, and his bowel movements were slightly loose. The thin, greasy coating on his tongue had decreased. His vision remained unchanged.

We modified the formula by removing Jujubae Fructus *(dà zǎo)* and Zingiberis Rhizoma recens *(shēng jiāng)* and adding Zingiberis Rhizoma praeparatum *(páo jiāng)* 6g. I gave him six more packets.

THIRD VISIT: The vision in the patient's right eye had become clearer and his visual distortion was no longer as noticeable. His bowel movements were normal, and his essence-spirit had improved.

We again modified the formula by adding Puerariae Radix *(gé gēn)* 20g and Viticis Fructus *(màn jīng zǐ)* 10g. I advised the patient to keep taking this formula for an extended period of time.

After taking 18 packets of this formula he reported that his vision was clear and no longer distorted. Upon examination, his visual acuity was 20/20 and the diffuse retinal macular edema with round spots of oozing fluid seen previously had completely resolved. I advised him to take Tonify the Middle to Augment the Qi Pill *(bǔ zhōng yì qì wán)* combined with Six-Gentlemen Pill with Aucklandia and Amomum *(xiāng shā liù jūn zǐ wán)* for one month to consolidate the treatment effect. I followed him for three years and there was no recurrence during that time.

REFLECTIONS AND CLARIFICATIONS

PHYSICIAN A   When you accepted this patient for treatment, you observed the presence of fatigue, dizziness, poor appetite, slightly loose stools, pale red tongue with a thin, white, greasy coating and a moderate, weak pulse. You diagnosed him with a lack of coordination between the ascending and descending functions of the Spleen and Stomach, along with yin fire bearing damp turbidity flooding upward. You then treated him with Raise the Yang and Augment the Stomach Decoction *(shēng yáng yì wèi tāng)* to tonify the Spleen and raise the clear, harmonize the Stomach and direct the turbid downward, and drain and restrain yin fire. After 30 packets, you obtained a complete cure. This outcome illustrates that when treating a local organic disease, one must still consider the holistic perspective. Furthermore, that one should be persistent with the strategy and the formula.

PHYSICIAN B   My feeling is that it is not so much whether or not one has a holistic perspective, but more importantly, how to practically make use of that perspective. For example, previous physicians had tried treating this patient with formulas to enrich the Liver and Kidney, tonify qi and blood, dredge the Liver and support the Spleen, and clear heat and resolve dampness. They had not been restricted to a narrow range of formulas that are commonly used for ophthalmologic diseases. Is this not also having a holistic perspective?

DR. YU   I would agree that the previous physicians had a holistic perspective and also that we can find a theoretical basis for all of their treatment strategies. The reason this theoretical basis exists is that in Chinese medicine, each organ forms its own system and the eyes are intimately connected to each of them. For example, in Chapter 80 of the *Divine Pivot (Líng shū)* the connection to the Heart is discussed: "The eyes are the envoy of the Heart." In Chapter 4 of *Basic Questions (Sū wèn)* the Liver is mentioned: "The Liver's opening orifice is the eyes." In Chapter 10 of *Basic Questions (Sū wèn)* it also states that "When the Liver receives blood, there is sight." Chapter 17 of the *Divine Pivot (Líng shū)* goes on to say that "Liver qi pervades the eyes. When the Liver is harmonious, the eyes can differentiate the five colors." Chapter 30 of the *Divine Pivot (Líng shū)* highlights the relationship of the eyes and the Lung: "When there is severe qi loss, the eyes do not see clearly." Chapter 33 of the *Divine Pivot (Líng shū)* discusses the connection of the eyes to the Kidneys: "When the Sea of Marrow is insufficient, the eyes cannot see." In *Secrets from the Orchid Chamber (Lán shì mì cáng)*, the relationship between the Spleen and the eyes becomes evident:

> The essence qi of all the organs is gathered in by the Spleen and then linked upward to the eyes. The Spleen is the first of all the yin [organs.] The eyes are the gathering [place] of the blood vessels. When the Spleen is deficient, the essence qi of the five yin organs loses its management and it fails to return to the eyes.

Chapter 80 of the *Divine Pivot (Líng shū)* sums up by stating that "The essence qi of all the organs flows upward into the eyes and makes them clear."

To speak plainly, when viewed through the lens of the historical record and the objective standards of science, this discussion easily results in a feeling of doubt with regard to what is right and wrong. For a physician without a solid grounding in clinical training, it can be very difficult to achieve a practical effect by only using a holistic perspective.

PHYSICIAN B   For this type of eye disease, Dr. Chen commonly used Augmented Preserve Vistas Formula *(zhù jǐng wán jiā jiǎn fāng)* successfully and yet that formula was ineffective in this case. Why was that?

DR. YU   The formula that he used contained Broussonetiae Fructus *(chǔ shí zǐ)*, Cuscutae Semen *(tù sī zǐ)*, Leonuri Fructus *(chōng wèi zǐ)*, Chaenomelis Fructus *(mù guā)*, Coicis Semen *(yì yǐ rén)*, powdered Notoginseng Radix *(sān qī)*, Gigeriae galli Endothelium corneum *(jī nèi jīn)*, dry-fried Setariae (Oryzae) Fructus germinatus *(chǎo gǔ yá)*, dry-fried Hordei Fructus germinatus *(chǎo mài yá)*, Lycii Fructus *(gǒu qǐ zǐ)*, and Dioscoreae Rhizoma *(shān yào)*. Within this formula, there is a relatively equal balance between medicinal substances that enrich the Kidneys and nourish the Liver with those that awaken the Spleen and resolve dampness. This type of formula is specific to eye diseases in which there is exhaustion of the Liver and Kidneys combined with Spleen deficiency and accompanying dampness.

If this patient had not already tried this approach, upon first seeing him, I would have tried it. Fortunately, I was able to draw lessons from the past failures, reassess the patient's pattern, and break out of the traditional fixed modes of thinking. I also relied on the critical teaching that "the macula pertains to the Spleen" and so switched my approach to address the middle burner. Thus, I changed to Raise the Yang and Augment the Stomach Decoction *(shēng yáng yì wèi tāng)* from Li Dong-Yuan. This formula tonifies the Spleen and raises the clear with a large dosage of Astragali Radix *(huáng qí)*, Codonopsis Radix *(dǎng shēn)*, and Atractylodis macrocephalae Rhizoma *(bái zhú)*. These medicinal substances are accompanied by Pinelliae Rhizoma praeparatum *(zhì bàn xià)*, Poria *(fú líng)* and Citri reticulatae Pericarpium *(chén pí)*, which harmonize the Stomach and direct the turbid downward. These functions are supported by Bupleuri Radix *(chái hú)*, Saposhnikoviae Radix *(fáng fēng)*, Notopterygii Rhizoma seu Radix *(qiāng huó)*, and Angelicae pubescentis Radix *(dú huó)*, which prevail over dampness by raising yang and scattering wind. The assistants, Coptidis Rhizoma *(huáng lián)*, Alismatis Rhizoma *(zé xiè)*, and Paeoniae Radix alba *(bái sháo)*, clear and drain, and restrain yin fire.

After writing this prescription, I was not filled with a sense of certainty and I told the patient that this type of visual disturbance could be difficult to treat quickly. I suggested that he start with six packets, wait for changes in the general symptoms, and then we would see how to proceed.

I think about the outcome as follows. Because my thought process and pattern differentiation was correct, it made sense to stick with the treatment strategy and the formula. By the time of the third visit, I gained confidence in my decision to maintain the strategy and formula because his vision was slightly clearer and the visual distortion he had experienced was much less noticeable.

PHYSICIAN C   I know that in ophthalmologic diseases you emphasize a holistic perspective, and in the case above, you grasped the clinical picture through an examination of the systemic symptoms. However, in some cases, when the disease is relatively mild, the systemic symptoms may not be obvious or they may be absent all together. What do you suggest in those cases?

DR. YU   I will give you a case example and you can draw your own conclusions from it. More than ten years ago I treated a middle-aged man with high degree myopia. Because the patient's home was very far away, although the left nose-piece on his glasses had fallen off, he had not had the time to get a new pair. As a result, the right side of the glasses was exerting an unusual amount of pressure, and after about six months, he started to feel aching and distention in the right orbit. After finally replacing his glasses and applying a warm compress to the right orbit, the soreness and distention decreased. However, from then on, he could not read or write for more than 30 minutes at a time, because after that he would notice a distinct increase in aching and heaviness in his right orbit.

An ophthalmologic examination revealed that the exterior of the eye was fine, but the vitreous body was turbid. Furthermore, although fundoscopic examination revealed high degree myopia, no other abnormalities were observed. Because there were no particular treatment steps to take, he was only offered vitamins and the suggestion to reduce the time spent reading and writing, while being mindful of getting enough rest.

Because of this situation, he was forced to rely on Chinese herbs. In looking at the four examinations, the only remarkable symptom was the local feeling of aching and distention in the patient's right orbit; everything else was normal, as were the tongue and pulse. Pattern differentiation was indeed difficult.

Nonetheless, I made the decision to begin by tonifying the Liver and Kidney because of the constitutional factor represented by the presence of significant myopia. I selected Augmented Preserve Vistas Pill *(jiā jiǎn zhù jǐng wán)*,[15] which I had him take as a decoction. After more than ten packets, there was no effect. I then changed to formulas such as Lycium Fruit, Chrysanthemum, and Rehmannia Pill *(qǐ jú dì huáng wán)*, Improve Vision Pill with Rehmannia *(míng mù dì huáng wán)*, and Rambling Powder *(xiāo yáo sǎn)*, but over the course of several months achieved no positive change.

The patient then became quite agitated after hearing that his symptoms could be a prodrome associated with retinal detachment. I became ashamed and disgruntled about my lack of success. Right at that time I was attending a professional conference and I took the opportunity to ask a colleague for advice. He gave me a faint smile and said, "This case is the pattern treated with Augment the Qi and Increase Acuity Decoction *(yì qì cōng míng tāng)* from *Indispensable Tools for Pattern Treatment (Zhèng zhì zhǔn shéng)*. What's the difficulty?"

I suddenly realized with a deep sigh that although I had searched everywhere for the answer without any success, the answer ended up coming without any effort on my part. I returned home with a strong desire to employ this new formula, but the patient had grown tired of preparing decoctions and was only willing to take pills. I thought about the fact that Augment the Qi and Increase Acuity Decoction *(yì qì cōng míng tāng)* tonified the Spleen, raised the clear, and drained and restrained yin fire. These principles seemed to be derived from the same origin as the major strategies of Li Dong-Yuan and so I chose to give him Li Dong-Yuan's Tonify the Middle to Augment the Qi Decoction *(bǔ zhōng yì qì tāng)*, which was readily available in pill form. After finishing one box (containing ten large pills), the patient reported that the aching and distention in his right orbit had decreased. He was very happy, and after taking ten boxes (100 pills), his symptoms had completely resolved and his orbit had returned to normal.

....

15. This formula is from *Essential Subtleties on the Silver Sea (Yín hǎi jīng wēi)*: Plantaginis Semen *(chē qián zǐ)*, Angelicae sinensis Radix *(dāng guī)*, Rehmanniae Radix praeparata *(shú dì huáng)*, Lycii Fructus *(gǒu qǐ zǐ)*, Zanthoxyli Pericarpium *(huā jiāo)*, Broussonetiae Fructus *(chǔ shí zǐ)*, Schisandrae Fructus *(wǔ wèi zǐ)*, and Cuscutae Semen *(tù sī zǐ)*.

PHYSICIAN B   I am still unclear. Tonify the Middle to Augment the Qi Decoction *(bǔ zhōng yì qì tāng)* tonifies the Spleen and Stomach, raises the yang, and augments the qi. How can it address aching and distention in the orbit?

DR. YU   I remember at the time having the same thought. When I started thinking about Augment the Qi and Increase Acuity Decoction *(yì qì cōng míng tāng)* though, I had a sudden realization. The orbit pertains to the Spleen. The unusual pressure exerted on the area, because of the problem with his glasses, had damaged the local qi and blood. The damage to qi and blood resulted in a failure of the normal qi circulation in the area, which gave rise to aching and distention. Tonify the Middle to Augment the Qi Decoction *(bǔ zhōng yì qì tāng)* tonified and raised the Spleen qi so that it reached the eyes. When the Spleen qi became sufficient, then the blood also became sufficient. When the qi moved, then the blood also moved. In the *Art of War (Sūn zǐ bīng fǎ)* it states that "Ingenuity stems from a focused mind." However, in this case, sublime usage arose from a sarcastic remark from a colleague that resolved my confusion. Thinking over my years as a clinician, I have often dealt with intractable diseases. Frequently, when I have been wracking my brains and feeling that I am at my wits' end, I have sought help from teachers and colleagues. I have not been ashamed to ask questions and to remain open to insight. I believe now more than ever that in traveling the path of scholarship it is invaluable to unabashedly ask questions.

5.4.2 Diplopia

A case of diplopia for four months

An effective formula that I created

投之皆效的自拟方

■ **CASE HISTORY**

Patient: *40-year-old man*

The patient was a driver who was generally healthy. Four months previously, after a stretch in which he had to drive for 24 hours, he became extremely fatigued. He showered, got drunk, and passed out in his clothes. Upon awakening, his right eye felt distended and painful, its motion felt constrained, and he was seeing double. At the time he also experienced dizziness, headache, fever, dry mouth, and thirst. He received treatment with a modification of Honeysuckle and Forsythia Powder *(yín qiáo sǎn)*, which resolved the symptoms, except for those directly related to his eye. The physician investigated the right eye and discovered that the pupil had shifted toward the lateral canthus (exotropia). He transferred the patient to the Western ophthalmology department where he was diagnosed with right oculomotor nerve palsy and admitted to the hospital. After attempting treatment with anti-allergic, anti-viral, anti-spasmodic, anti-inflammatory and steroidal medications, all of which were ineffective, they felt that there was no alternative but to try Chinese herbs.

The first physician diagnosed him as having a wind pathogen that directly struck the channels and collaterals. He prescribed a modification of Minor Extend Life Decoction *(xiǎo xù mìng tāng)*. After taking one packet, the distention and pain in the patient's eye increased, and he reported dizziness, irritability, restlessness, and dry mouth. The next physician consulted diagnosed him with yin deficiency and hyperactive yang and prescribed a modification of Gastrodia and Uncaria Drink *(tiān má gōu téng yǐn)*. After eight packets, all the systemic symptoms had decreased in severity, but the abnormality of the patient's right eye remained unchanged. The formula was made into pills and it was suggested that he continue taking it, alternating with Lycium Fruit, Chrysanthemum, and Rehmannia Pill *(qǐ jú dì huáng wán)*, Improve Vision Pill with Rehmannia *(míng mù dì huáng wán)*, Dendrobium Pill for Night Vision *(shí hú yè guāng wán)*, and Magnetite and Cinnabar Pill *(cí zhū wán)*. However, after more than two months of this approach, his symptoms persisted.

INTAKE EXAMINATION
NOVEMBER 13, 1992

The patient was experiencing diplopia and felt that his right eye was slightly distended. Exotropia was observed and eye motion constrained (not fluid). He also reported dry mouth and constipation. His tongue was pale red, lacked moisture, and had a scanty coating. His pulse was wiry and fine.

DIFFERENTIATION OF PATTERNS AND DISCUSSION OF TREATMENT

PHYSICIAN A In the tradition of Chinese medicine, ophthalmology divides eye disorders into two broad categories of disease: internal and external obstructions. To which category does this case belong?

DR. YU Neither. Ophthalmology in contemporary Chinese medicine places this case in the general category of 'other eye diseases,' specifically 'vision pulled to one side by wind.' The special characteristics of this disease are that it has a sudden onset and manifests with deviation of the pupil and diplopia. When the disease is severe, classical Chinese literature categorizes this pattern as wind striking the channels and collaterals. The pattern is referred to as "eye deviation from wind" by Wei Yi-Lin in his Yuan-dynasty text, *Effective Formulas from Generations of Physicians (Shì yī dé xiào fāng)*. In the modern reference work *Concise Dictionary of Chinese Medicine (Jiǎn míng zhōng yī cí diǎn)*, eye deviation from wind is described as follows:

> lax closure of the eyelid (or, in severe cases, lower lid eversion), deviated eyeball, the patient's cheek and lips deviate to one side, and he or she may experience involuntary tremors. This condition may be accompanied by dizziness, diplopia, red eyes, involuntary tearing, and in severe cases, hemiplegia.

This describes an acute episode of severe facial paralysis and many areas can be affected. In the case described above, the symptoms of diplopia, deviation of the eyeball, and constrained eye motion are seen locally around the eye. Thus, the diagnosis of 'vision pulled to one side by wind' is accurate.

Treatment and Outcome

We considered this to be exhausted Liver yin and phlegm obstructing the collaterals. The appropriate treatment was to enrich Liver yin, transform phlegm, dispel stasis, and unblock the collaterals. We decided to try a somewhat awkward formula that I had created called Decoction to Nourish the Liver and Unblock the Collaterals (yǎng gān tōng luò tāng):

Mume Fructus (wū méi)	15g
Polygoni cuspidati Rhizoma (hǔ zhàng)	30g
Ziziphi spinosae Semen (suān zǎo rén)	15g
Paeoniae Radix alba (bái sháo)	15g
charred Rehmanniae Radix (shēng dì huáng tàn)	30g
charred Toosendan Fructus (chuān liàn zǐ tàn)	6g
Glehniae Radix (běi shā shēn)	20g
Ophiopogonis Radix (mài mén dōng)	20g
Lycii Fructus (gǒu qǐ zǐ)	15g
Glycyrrhizae Radix praeparata (zhì gān cǎo)	6g
Bombyx Batryticatus (bái jiāng cán)	10g
Pheretima (dì lóng)	10g
Persicae Semen (táo rén)	6g

We instructed the patient to take ten packets and to cease taking all other medicinal substances, Chinese or Western.

Second Visit: After having taken ten packets of the formula he reported positive progress. The right eyeball was only occasionally distended, the eye deviation was less, the eye moved more smoothly and easily, and the diplopia had improved. He no longer had a dry mouth and his bowel movements were smooth.

Because the formula was effective, I made no changes. He continued with 15 more packets of the formula. After taking them, his vision had completely returned to normal and all the accompanying symptoms had resolved. Follow-up at one year revealed no recurrence.

Disease	Primary symptoms	Differential diagnosis	Treatment method	Formula
Vision pulled to one side by wind	Diplopia, deviated pupil, jerky motion of the eyeball	Exhaustion and deficiency of the Liver yin; phlegm and stasis obstructing the collaterals	Enrich and nourish the Liver yin, transform phlegm, expel stasis, and open up the collaterals	Decoction to Nourish the Liver and Unblock the Collaterals (yǎng gān tōng luò tāng)

Reflections and Clarifications

PHYSICIAN B   How do you understand the etiology and pathodynamic of 'vision pulled to one side by wind'?

DR. YU   Chapter 80 of the Divine Pivot (Líng shū) states that "The essence qi of the yin and yang organs pours upward into the eyes and makes them clear." In general, when the essence qi of the organs is exhausted, sudden attack of wind causes this disease. It can also be caused by external trauma to the eye. Contemporary textbooks on Chinese ophthalmology divide this disease into four patterns: exterior invasion of wind-heat that directly attacks the channels and collaterals; Spleen qi deficiency with phlegm-dampness obstructing the collaterals; qi and blood deficiency with pathogenic wind invasion; and insufficiency of the true source with wind and fire rising.

Clinically, what we observe is that overwork and prolonged use of the eyes depletes Liver blood and harms Liver yin. Then wind attacks and causes this disease. This etiology is the most common one and it is what we observe in the case above.

PHYSICIAN C   Your explanation certainly seems reasonable from the perspective of Chinese medicine, but it seems overly general and abstract. Would it be possible for you to explain specifically why in this case the patient experienced diplopia?

DR. YU   For a specific explanation, we use Western medicine as a reference. According to Western ophthalmology, diplopia is the result of an irregularity in the movements of the extraocular muscles.[16] No matter which way the eyeball moves, all 12 of the extraocular muscles must work in concert to insure that the image is projected onto the retina correctly. Only then can the processing of the visual cortex create a single image from the two eyes. Thus, irregular movement of the extraocular muscles can produce diplopia. In the final analysis, irregular movement of the extraocular muscles is actually the result of nerve paralysis in the relevant nerves: the oculomotor nerve (3rd cranial nerve), trochlear nerve (4th cranial nerve) and abducens nerve (6th cranial nerve). In the present case, diplopia resulted from paralysis of the oculomotor nerve causing dysfunction of the medial rectus muscle.

Although this explanation is concrete and accurate, nonetheless, pharmaceutical treatment is often insufficient to treat the problem and some patients end up resorting to surgery, which often creates its own problems. In some of these cases, it turns out that treatment with Chinese herbal medicine can be quite helpful.

PHYSICIAN A   What strategies and formulas are frequently used for 'vision pulled to one side by wind'?

DR. YU   I make the decision about treatment on the basis of the level of urgency, symptom intensity, and duration of the disease. For example, if the disease is acute onset wind-heat directly attacking the channels and collaterals in an otherwise healthy patient, presenting with symptoms such as fever, chills, and headache, Minor Extend Life Decoction *(xiǎo xù mìng tāng)* should be used to dispel wind and unblock the collaterals.

For patients with a constitutional insufficiency of true yin, when emotional provocation such as recurrent troubles, losing one's temper, or panic produces hyperactivity of Liver yang, wind stirring, and phlegm obstruction, it can produce a relatively severe and urgent situation with symptoms such as dizziness and instability, numbness, contractions, and tremors, and in severe cases a drooping eyelid and a deviated mouth. This situation should be addressed with the combination of Gastrodia and Uncaria Drink *(tiān má gōu téng yǐn)* and Sedate the Liver and Extinguish Wind Decoction *(zhèn gān xī fēng tāng)* to calm the Liver and anchor the yang, and to transform phlegm and unblock the collaterals.

....
16. *Translators' note:* There are six extraocular muscles on each side: medial rectus, lateral rectus, superior rectus, inferior oblique, superior oblique, and ciliary.

In my experience, in cases with acute onset, even when severe, if the treatment is timely and the formula is correct, you can often eliminate or significantly ameliorate the presenting symptoms. However, if there is deviation of the eye and diplopia, these symptoms are typically difficult to resolve in a short period of time. In these cases, it is important to make a deliberate plan, considering the pathodynamic and relevant constitutional factors.

In cases where the pattern is one of Spleen qi deficiency with phlegm-dampness obstructing the collaterals, fortify the Spleen, augment the qi, dispel wind and phlegm, and unblock the collaterals with a combination of Tonify the Middle to Augment the Qi Decoction (bǔ zhōng yì qì tāng) and Correct the Appearance Decoction (zhèng róng tāng).[17] If there is injury to Liver yin with phlegm and stasis obstructing the collaterals, nourish Liver yin, transform phlegm, dispel stasis, and unblock the collaterals with a modification of either Rehmannia Pill (dì zhī wán)[18] or Preserve Vistas Pill (zhù jǐng wán). Over the years in my clinical experience, there have been some cases that did not respond well to any of these treatment strategies and I have had no alternative but to try my own formula, Decoction to Nourish the Liver and Unblock the Collaterals (yǎng gān tōng luò tāng). In the more than ten cases in which I have used this formula, it has yielded reasonably satisfactory results.

PHYSICIAN B   The formula you created seems to have emerged from your frequent use of Linking Decoction (yī guàn jiān). Why did you feel the need to give it a separate name?

DR. YU   Although the ingredients in my formula are certainly related to those in Wei Liu-Zhou's Linking Decoction (yī guàn jiān), the strategy and formula structure are more in line with the thinking of Zhang Zhong-Jing. In *Essentials from the Golden Cabinet (Jīn guì yào lüè)*, it states that, "In Liver disease, tonify with sour [flavors], assist with charred and bitter [flavors], augment with sweet flavors to adjust it." It further clarifies, "When the Liver is deficient, use this strategy, but when it is excessive, do not use it." My formulation relies on the sour, restraining actions of Mume Fructus (wū méi), Ziziphi spinosae Semen (suān zǎo rén), Polygoni cuspidati Rhizoma (hǔ zhàng), and Paeoniae Radix alba (bái sháo), in conjunction with the sweet, moderate actions of Glehniae Radix (běi shā shēn), Ophiopogonis Radix (mài mén dōng), Lycii Fructus (gǒu qǐ zǐ), and Glycyrrhizae Radix praeparata (zhì gān cǎo) to nourish Liver yin. The charred, bitter flavors of charred Rehmanniae Radix (shēng dì huáng tàn) and charred Toosendan Fructus (chuān liàn zǐ tàn) drain Liver fire and shield Liver yin. The combination of Bombyx Batryticatus (bái jiāng cán), Pheretima (dì lóng), and Persicae Semen (táo rén) transforms phlegm, dispels stasis, and unblocks the collaterals.

....

17. Correct the Appearance Decoction (zhèng róng tāng) comes from *Scrutiny of the Precious Jade Case (Shěn shì yáo hán)*, an ophthalmology text written by Fu Ren-Yu and published in 1642. It contains Notopterygii Rhizoma seu Radix (qiāng huó), Typhonii Rhizoma praeparatum (zhì bái fù zǐ), Saposhnikoviae Radix (fáng fēng), Gentianae macrophyllae Radix (qín jiāo), Arisaema cum Bile (dǎn nán xīng), Bombyx Batryticatus (bái jiāng cán), Pinelliae Rhizoma praeparatum (zhì bàn xià), Chaenomelis Fructus (mù guā), Glycyrrhizae Radix (gān cǎo), and Poriae Sclerotium pararadicis (fú shén mù)

18. Rehmannia Pill (dì zhī wán) contains Rehmanniae Radix (shēng dì huáng), Asparagi Radix (tiān mén dōng), Aurantii Fructus (zhǐ ké), and Chrysanthemi Flos (jú huā)

It is worth noting that from a Western ophthalmologic perspective, the patho-dynamic of this disease is nerve paralysis that results in a lack of coordinated move-ment in the extraocular muscles. From a Chinese medicine perspective, the extraocular muscles are considered to 'bind and tie.' My notion is that irregularity in the binding and tying function of the eyes is most likely the responsibility of the Liver, specifically the Liver functions of dredging, draining, and thrusting out. If my notion is not too absurd, then when considering appropriate treatment, it makes sense to greatly enrich Liver yin while simultaneously assisting by dredging the Liver and dispersing constraint. This formula does not contain special ingredients for dredging the Liver and dispersing constraint, instead it relies on Mume Fructus *(wū méi)* and Polygoni cuspidati Rhizo-ma *(hǔ zhàng)*, each of which has a strong unblocking force contained within its sour, restraining actions.

PHYSICIAN B   According to all of the major materia medica, Polygoni cuspidati Rhizoma *(hǔ zhàng)* is bitter and cold. Its actions are described as invigorating blood and settling pain, clearing heat and resolving dampness, resolving toxicity, and transforming phlegm and stopping cough. What is the basis for your assertion that it is sour and restraining, while also opening and unblocking?

DR. YU   In rural Sichuan, Polygonum cuspidatum *(hǔ zhàng)* is known by the peasants as speckled bamboo (花斑竹 *huā bān zhú*). The fresh plant is sour and very juicy. Peas-ant children pick the stalks and chew them to release the juice. The *Comprehensive Outline of the Materia Medica (Běn cǎo gāng mù)* notes that peasants pick the roots, wash them clean, and cook them with Glycyrrhizae Radix *(gān cǎo)*. The resulting liquid is sour, sweet, and used as a cooling drink in the summertime. My teacher, Jian Yu-Guang, who is in his 80s, was originally a traveling doctor in western Sichuan. He gained wide renown for his treatment of Liver disease, and the primary ingredient in his secret formulas was Polygoni cuspidati Rhizoma *(hǔ zhàng)*. He said "Polygoni cuspidati Rhizoma *(hǔ zhàng)* enriches Liver yin, dredges the Liver, and disperses constraint. It is so good at this that its function surpasses Mume Fructus *(wū méi)*."

There is some support for this view in the earlier materia medicae. The 6th-century work *Miscellaneous Records of Famous Physicians (Míng yī bié lù)* notes that Polygoni cuspidati Rhizoma *(hǔ zhàng)* "unblocks menstruation, and breaks up retained blood and fixed abdominal masses." The 8th-century *Materia Medica of Ri Hua-Zi (Rì Huá-Zǐ běn cǎo)* states that Polygoni cuspidati Rhizoma *(hǔ zhàng)* "treats postpartum failure of noxious blood to descend, and distention and fullness in the epigastrium and abdomen, it expels pus … [treats] harm from static blood, and breaks up wind toxin and knotted qi." Is that not a textual reference supporting the ability of Polygoni cuspidati Rhizoma *(hǔ zhàng)* to 'open and unblock'?

In my experience of treating habitual constipation, when I add a large dosage of Polygoni cuspidati Rhizoma *(hǔ zhàng)* to whatever appropriate formula I am using, the results are even quicker. Even using Polygoni cuspidati Rhizoma *(hǔ zhàng)* by itself for constipation is effective. Is this not 'opening and unblocking'? A philosopher has said that all knowledge in the world originates with direct personal experience. This is certainly true.

PHYSICIAN C   In this case you described making the decision to "try out" Decoction to Nourish the Liver and Unblock the Collaterals *(yǎng gān tōng luò tāng)* to treat the eye pulled to one side by wind. Is it true that this formula can also be used to treat other diseases?

DR. YU   This formula can be used very broadly to treat symptoms such as headache, dizziness, vertigo, hypochondriac pain, heartburn, indefinable epigastric discomfort, numbness of the extremities, and deficiency-type constipation, as long as they belong to a pattern of exhausted Liver yin and phlegm obstructing the collaterals. It can be effective for all of these conditions.

Appendix

Time and Space in Chinese Medical Therapeutics

Treat winter diseases in summer and summer diseases in winter

冬病夏治,夏病冬治

■ CASE HISTORY NO. 1

Patient: *56-year-old man*

The patient had chronic bronchitis for over 20 years and his general constitution has become worse in recent years. While in the summer he was basically all right, once autumn arrived he would become worried as he easily felt cold, coughed up profuse sputum, and his breathing became tight. Both Western and Chinese medicines had been tried, but the disorder was recalcitrant and proved difficult to cure. When the season turned to winter the patient became prone to pulmonary infections that necessitated a stay in the hospital that included intravenous medications.

INTAKE EXAMINATION

At the time of the exam his chronic bronchitis had flared into an acute bronchitis with associated infection and he had already been in the hospital for 20 days and been treated by multiple types of antibiotics along with Chinese medicines. While the infection was under control, he still had a cough with stagnant sputum, tight breathing, reduced intake, and unformed stools. His tongue body was washed-out, the coating was thin, greasy, and white, and his pulse weak.

■ CASE HISTORY NO. 2

Patient: *26-year-old woman*

This woman was born prematurely and as a child was weak and often ill. Since the age of five she had a cough that lasted 2-3 months every summer. During these episodes her throat was itchy, which led to a hacking, non-productive cough. At the height of summer her hacking coughs became even more intense.

Every year as soon as the coughing began she hurried to get treatment with such things as IVs and oral medicine, but these only provided temporary relief and the problem frequently recurred. With the onset of autumnal coolness the coughing would become less frequent, and would occur even more rarely after the winter solstice when the temperature was at its coldest.

This year she came to see me one month after the onset of the coughing.

INTAKE EXAMINATION

She is thin with an ashen complexion and very dry skin. When her throat becomes itchy she will start on coughing jags that will last from a dozen to many dozens of coughs. Only after she has coughed up some very sticky sputum will the coughing temporarily halt. She has a dry mouth and likes to drink fluids. She has yellow urine, dry stools, and a tongue that is tender and red with a patchy and peeling coat (geographic tongue). Her pulse is wiry, big, and lacks force.

DIFFERENTIATION OF PATTERNS AND DISCUSSION OF TREATMENT

DR. YU   These patients' problems are either more severe in the winter and milder in the summer, or more severe in the summer and milder in the winter. When more severe in the winter, they have a yang deficient constitution; when more severe in the summer, they have a yin deficient constitution. These two types of characteristic constitutions from yin/yang biases were present in ancient times. As it states in Chapter 64 of the *Divine Pivot (Līng shū)*, some people "can endure spring and summer and cannot endure autumn and winter;" others "can endure autumn and winter and cannot endure spring and summer."

This leads us to consider one of the singular treatment methods in Chinese medicine—treating winter-time diseases in summer and summer-time diseases in winter. A preliminary survey would indicate that this approach is appropriate for debilitating diseases that are more severe in one set of seasons and milder in the other. While these approaches are discussed as being a method for treating disease, it would be better if they were discussed as methods for *treating constitutions*. That is, once the constitution has been improved and strengthened it will be restored to a healthy state. As stated in Chapter 3 of *Basic Questions (Sù wèn)*, "When the yin is balanced and the yang sealed, the essence and spirit are in order." There is nothing mysterious about this; it is nothing more than a means of treating disease before it manifests.

PHYSICIAN A   The idea put forward in the *Inner Classic (Nèi jīng)* that the superior practitioner "treats when there is not yet a disease" is explained in modern textbooks as the three aspects: "early prevention when there is no disease," "early treatment when there is a disease," and "prepare for changes when there is a full-on disease." If it is like this, then wouldn't "treating when there is not yet a disease" be accomplished by tonifying the yang in the winter when the yang qi is especially deficient, and tonifying the yin in summer when the yin essence is especially deficient?

DR. YU   "Treating when there is not yet a disease" is found in Chapter 2 of the *Basic Questions (Sù wèn)*, which is a chapter describing how humans should live in sync with the seasons—generating life in spring, growing in summer, harvesting in autumn, and storing in winter in accordance with the laws of nature. This nourishes life and prevents disease, and if you turn your back on these laws of nature, illness will come. As the original text stated, "Going against [these laws] leads to disaster and harms life; following them, not even minor illnesses will arise." This leads to the famous dictum, "The sages did not treat those who were already ill, but treated those who were not yet ill."

From this we can see that "treating when there is not yet a disease" indeed has the connotation of doing early preventative work when a disease has not yet occurred, such as nourishing life to ward off disease. Yet clearly "early treatment when there is a disease" is not treating when there is not yet a disease. Now, let us address "prepare for changes when there is a full-on disease." This is like what Zhang Zhong-Jing noted in the first chapter of the *Essentials from the Golden Cabinet (Jīn guì yò lüè)*: "When one sees a disease of the Liver, know that the Liver will transmit it to the Spleen, so first bolster the Spleen." This is treating the organ that has not yet become diseased, and while this is an extension of the concept expressed in the *Inner Classic (Nèi jīng)*, in the end it does not qualify as an example of treating when there is not yet a disease.

How can we finally understand early prevention and what it means to truly treat a disease that has not yet developed? Chapter 2 of the *Basic Questions (Sù wèn)* states, "During spring and summer nourish the yang, during autumn and winter nourish the yin." My understanding of this passage is that for people with balanced and harmonious yin and yang, one should emphasize nourishing and protecting of the yang-qi in the spring and summer and the yin-essence in the autumn and winter. Transferring this way of nourishing life into the framework of Chinese medical therapeutics, we can conclude that one should warm the yang in summer for winter diseases and enrich the yin in winter for summer diseases. This is not the facile understanding of this concept that most people harbor that "One should tonify the yang in winter when the yang qi is especially deficient and tonify the yin in summer when the yin essence is especially deficient."

PHYSICIAN B   I have read quite a bit about your experiences treating winter diseases in summer and summer diseases in winter. In summer, in addition to using Restore the Right [Kidney] Pill *(yòu guī wán)*, you have also used formulas that warm the yang, such as Aconite Accessory Root Pill to Regulate the Middle *(fù zǐ lǐ zhōng wán)*, Balmy Yang Decoction *(yáng hé tāng)*, Cinnamon Twig plus Aconite Accessory Root Decoction *(guì zhī jiā fù zǐ tāng)*, and yang-warming substances like Hominis Placenta *(zǐ hé chē)* and Cervi Cornu pantotrichum *(lù róng)*. In winter, besides Restore the Left [Kidney] Pill *(zuǒ guī wán)*, you have also used approaches that enrich the yin, such as Great Tonify the Yin Pill *(dà bǔ yīn wán)*, Enrich Water and Clear the Liver Drink *(zī shuǐ qīng gān yǐn)*, Linking Decoction *(yī guàn jiān)*, and yin-enriching substances like Testudinis Plastrum *(guī bǎn)* and Asini Corii Colla *(ē jiāo)*.

Despite these formulas and herbs being chosen when it is not their supposed time, not only has their use not provoked any side effects, but they have had a definite effect, sometimes with rather good results.

TREATMENT AND OUTCOME

■ CASE HISTORY NO. 1

Winter disease treated in summer

The diagnosis was qi deficiency of the Lung and Spleen with the Lung losing its ability to disseminate and clarify. The patient was given six packets of a modified combination of Six-Gentlemen Decoction *(liù jūn zǐ tāng)* and Inula Powder *(jīn fèi cǎo sǎn)* after which all the symptoms had decreased. This was followed by ten packets of a combination of Ginseng, Poria, and White Atractylodes Powder *(shēn líng bái zhú sǎn)* and Tonify the Middle to Augment the Qi Decoction *(bǔ zhōng yì qì tāng)*, which he took home upon being discharged from the hospital.

Before leaving the hospital, the patient came to see me about how to treat his chronic bronchitis. Being deeply worried, he inquired about treatment and prevention approaches to chronic bronchitis saying, "Every autumn I fall ill, approaching winter is like entering the gates of hell. My body is increasingly weak, and I fear I may not live to the age of 60."

I gave him a quick explanation of Chinese medicine's view on nourishing life and also suggested that he try summer-time treatment of winter diseases. This made him quite happy.

I then gave him the following prescription of Restore the Right [Kidney] Pill *(yòu guī wán)*, Ginseng and Walnut Decoction *(rén shēn hú táo tāng)*, and Ginseng and Gecko Powder *(rén shēn gé jiè sǎn)* with some additions:

Rehmanniae Radix praeparata *(shú dì huáng)*	400g
Dioscoreae Rhizoma *(shān yào)*	200g
Corni Fructus *(shān zhū yú)*	100g
Lycii Fructus *(gǒu qǐ zǐ)*	150g
Cuscutae Semen *(tù sī zǐ)*	150g
Cervi Cornus Colla *(lù jiǎo jiāo)*	150g
dry-fried Eucommiae Cortex *(chǎo dù zhòng)*	150g
Cinnamomi Cortex *(ròu guì)*	100g
Angelicae sinensis Radix *(dāng guī)*	100g
Aconiti Radix lateralis praeparata *(zhì fù zǐ)*	100g
Ginseng Radix rubra *(hóng shēn)*	100g
Juglandis Semen *(hé táo rén)*	100g
Gecko *(gé jiè)*	30g
Fritillariae cirrhosae Bulbus *(chuān bèi mǔ)*	30g
Hominis Placenta *(zǐ hé chē)*	60g
dry-fried Hordei Fructus germinatus *(chǎo mài yá)*	200g

METHOD OF PREPARATION: Place the ingredients in an oven and bake until crisp. Then grind them into a fine powder and make into pills with refined honey, with each pill being about 15g. Place the pills in a refrigerator for cold storage.

METHOD OF ADMINISTRATION: Starting on the day of the summer solstice, make a daily infusion of 30g each of Astragali Radix (huáng qí), Agrimoniae Herba (xiān hè cǎo), and Epimedii Herba (yín yáng huò) and take one pill with this infusion. Continue administrating until the day of the end of summerheat (處暑 chǔ shǔ) [this is the 14th of 24 solar terms in the Chinese calendar and usually falls in early September]. The patient should stop taking this medicine when they have a cold.

FOLLOW-UP

The patient took the above medicine for three months and followed the method of administration. While that year he still had frequent bouts of coughing and wheezing, they were milder than in previous years, and every time it was controlled by a number of packets of herbs based on a combination of Apricot Kernel and Perilla Leaf Powder (xìng sū sǎn) and Stop Coughing Powder (zhǐ sòu sǎn). Only at the end of [the 23rd solar term] minor cold (小寒 xiǎo hán) did he contract a pulmonary infection that required a 10-day stay in the hospital.

The next year he continued with the same formula and method of administration and his constitution improved. In the fall his bouts of coughing were infrequent and he used a modified version of Apricot Kernel and Perilla Leaf Powder (xìng sū sǎn) and Stop Coughing Powder (zhǐ sòu sǎn) intermittently for them. In winter when the coughing and wheezing became more severe, he was seen as an outpatient and treated successfully with intravenous medications and Chinese herbs. He was not admitted to the hospital any time during that year. He continued in this fashion for five years and his constitution clearly grew more robust, his complexion ruddy, and he rarely became ill.

■ CASE HISTORY NO. 2

Summer disease treated in winter

The diagnosis was yin exhaustion of the Spleen and Lung such that the fluids did not moisten the throat. She was given a modified combination of Generate the Pulse Powder (shēng mài sǎn) and Six Ingredient Laryngology Decoction (hóu kē liù wèi tāng):[1]

Glehniae Radix (běi shā shēn)	15g
Pseudostellariae Radix (tài zǐ shēn)	15g
Ophiopogonis Radix (mài mén dōng)	15g
Schisandrae Fructus (wǔ wèi zǐ)	10g
Schizonepetae Herba (jīng jiè)	5g
Platycodi Radix (jié gěng)	6g
Glycyrrhizae Radix praeparata (zhì gān cǎo)	6g
Menthae haplocalycis Herba (bò hé)	6g

....
1. For more information on this formula, see pp. 25-6 of *A Walk Along the River*.

Cicadae Periostracum *(chán tuì)*... 10g

Belamcandae Rhizoma *(shè gān)*.. 10g

prepared Stemonae Radix *(zhì bǎi bù)*.................................... 10g

Bombyx batryticatus *(bái jiāng cán)* 10g

After taking six packets, the patient's throat itching and hacking cough had diminished. Schizonepetae Herba *(jīng jiè)* and Menthae haplocalycis Herba *(bò hé)* were removed and 30g of Dioscoreae Rhizoma *(shān yào)* and 10g of Arctii Fructus *(niú bàng zǐ)* were added. After taking another six packets of this modified prescription, the throat itching and hacking cough had stopped. However, they recurred in less than a couple of weeks.

At this time the original formula was used again and it was suggested that the following be used as a form of treating summer diseases in the winter:

Rehmanniae Radix *(shēng dì huáng)*............................. 400g

Dioscoreae Rhizoma *(shān yào)* 200g

Corni Fructus *(shān zhū yú)*... 200g

Achyranthis bidentatae Radix *(niú xī)* 150g

dry-fried pearls of Testudinis Plastri Colla *(guī bǎn jiāo, chǎo zhū)*...... 200g

Gecko *(gé jiè)*... 30g

Panacis quinquefolii Radix *(xī yáng shēn)*..................... 30g

Fritillariae cirrhosae Bulbus *(chuān bèi mǔ)*.................. 30g

Juglandis Semen *(hé táo rén)* 30g

Glehniae Radix *(běi shā shēn)* 200g

Ophiopogonis Radix *(mài mén dōng)* 200g

Paeoniae Radix alba *(bái sháo)*.................................... 200g

Glycyrrhizae Radix praeparata *(zhì gān cǎo)* 100g

dry-fried Hordei Fructus germinatus *(chǎo mài yá)* 200g

METHOD OF PREPARATION: Place the ingredients in an oven and bake until crisp. Then grind them into a fine powder and make into pills with refined honey, with each pill being about 15g. Place the pills in a refrigerator for cold storage.

METHOD OF ADMINISTRATION: Starting on the day of the winter solstice, make an infusion every day of 30g each of Ecliptae Herba *(mò hàn lián)*, Agrimoniae Herba *(xiān hè cǎo)*, and Epimedii Herba *(yín yáng huò)* and take one pill with this infusion before each meal. Continue administrating until the day of the vernal equinox (春分 *chūn fèn*) [this is the fourth of 24 solar terms in the Chinese calendar and usually falls in late March]. The patient should stop taking this medicine when they have a cold.

FOLLOW-UP

The patient took the above medicine as directed for three months, and the next summer, while she still had a hacking cough, it was milder and stopped after taking ten packets of the modified combination of Generate the Pulse Powder *(shēng mài sǎn)* and Six Ingredient Laryngology Decoction *(hóu kē liù wèi tāng)*. There was a relapse, but the total time she was sick was less than a full month. She continued to take the winter-time formula for three years, as described above. After this the hacking cough that had bothered her for 20 years did not recur.

REFLECTIONS AND CLARIFICATIONS

PHYSICIAN A   When you say that in those whose problems are worse in the winter and milder in the summer have a yang deficient constitution and those whose problems are worse in the summer and milder in the winter have a yin deficient constitution, that is easy to understand. Yet from another perspective, as the weather during winter is frigid cold, at this time those with a deficient yang constitution should become even more deficient; and as the weather during the summer is blazingly hot, at that time those with a deficient yin constitution should become even more deficient. Therefore, it is reasonable to have it laid out like this:

- those with a yang deficient constitution should have their yang qi warmed and tonified during the winter to resist the intense winter cold;

- those with a yin deficient constitution should have their yin essence enriched and nourished during the summer to resist the blazing summer heat.

The formulas and herbs that you suggest are used in exactly the opposite manner: in summer use those that warm the yang, as in Restore the Right [Kidney] Pill *(yòu guī wán)* in Case no. 1 above, and in winter use those that enrich the yin, as in Restore the Left [Kidney] Pill *(zǔo guī wán)* in Case no. 2 above.

DR. YU   Let me give an example. Once a young Chinese doctor thought:

> A year has four seasons—spring/warmth, summer/heat, autumn/coolness, and winter/cold. These all are natural phenomena. Human beings have become accustomed to using the cold to escape the summer heat by drinking heat-clearing and cooling drinks and in winter using warmth to escape the cold by eating warming and tonifying things (as in the extra tonics taken around the winter solstice).

This viewpoint represents that of the majority of the general population. However, to me these customs clearly go against Chinese medicine's approach to nourishing life.

You don't believe me? Let's look at a true story about this young Chinese doctor. In the summer of 1968 he drank an infusion of 5g Ilicis latifoliae Folium *(kǔ dīng chá)* daily and gradually developed a full and stifling sensation in his stomach. As he continued drinking this infusion for three months, his appetite gradually declined, food lost its taste, his stools became loose, and he developed profuse nocturia.

He realized that his Spleen had been harmed and took Regulate the Middle Pill *(lǐ zhōng wán)*, but to no avail. He then came asking for help to my first teacher, Jian Yu-Guang. Dr. Jian gave him six packets of Aconite Accessory Root Decoction to Regulate the Middle *(fù zǐ lǐ zhōng wán)*, adding 1.5g of Sulfur *(liú huáng)* to each dose. The symptoms gradually subsided, but for several years after that, he would again develop a stifling and full sensation in his epigastrium, and loose stools, if he ate even a small amount of melons, fruit, or other raw-cold items. This shows that for those with a yang deficient constitution, eating cold things in summer will just make a bad situation worse. It is like adding frost on top of snow.

PHYSICIAN B   However, I respectfully submit that these views can be refuted. The Tang-dynasty writer Wang Bing annotated the passage, "In spring and summer nourish the yang; in autumn and winter nourish the yin" from Chapter 2 of the *Basic Questions (Sù wèn)*, taking "nourish" (養 *yǎng*) as "control" (制 *zhì*), advocating eating cool food in spring and cold food in summer to control the yang, and eating warm food in autumn and hot food in winter to control the yin. The famous Ming-dynasty author Li Shi-Zhen wrote in his *Comprehensive Outline of the Materia Medica (Běn cǎo gāng mù)*, "Eat cool foods in spring and cold foods sin summer to nourish the yang; eat warm foods in autumn and hot foods in winter to nourish the yin." Can it be that these prominent figures in Chinese medicine all were mistaken?

PHYSICIAN C   Cold and cool things easily damage the yang-qi and warm and hot things easily damage the yin-fluids. Wang's annotation flies in the face of what is common knowledge in Chinese medicine. Still, Wang's annotations had a non-negligible influence on later generations. Li Shi-Zhen is not alone in following his explanations, as there are even contemporary physicians who believe this. Dr. Yu, you have long disagreed with Wang's annotation and wrote an essay to that effect in an academic dispute with true believers on this issue in the journal *Shaanxi Chinese Medicine* in 1982.

DR. YU   When I was younger and came across Wang's annotation while studying the *Basic Questions (Sù wèn)*, I was quite suspicious of it and so asked my mentor, Dr. Jian Yu-Guang. Dr. Jian grinned and said that Wang's annotation misled people. I questioned Dr. Jian, asking if those with a yang deficient constitution really can't tolerate cold and cool foods. "If that is the case," I probed, "in Chapter 25 of the *Basic Questions (Sù wèn)* it says, 'Humans come to life through the qi of heaven and earth.' Humans also live as small versions of heaven and earth. As during the summer the yang qi of heaven and earth are abundant and flourishing, how can it be that we cannot tolerate cold and cool things?" Dr. Jian replied that during the scorching heat of summer, the water in wells is cool, and in the frigid cold of winter, the water in wells is warm. This shows that in summer when the yang of heaven is abundant, the yang of earth is deficient; in winter when the yin of heaven is abundant, the yin of earth is deficient. Humans are placed between heaven and earth where their qi intersects, so in summer the external yang is abundant while the internal yang is deficient; in winter the external yin is abundant while the internal yin is deficient.

PHYSICIAN B   Dr. Jian's explanation uses correspondences extremely well. It is simple, yet profound, as well as enlightening. Does the literature include anything like it?

DR. YU   It does. Later I read *Collected Annotations on the Yellow Emperor's Inner Classic: Basic Questions (Huáng Dì nèi jīng sù wèn jí zhù)* by the 17th-century author Zhang Zhi-Cong. When I got to his annotation of "in spring and summer nourish the yang; in autumn and winter nourish the yin," I couldn't help but clap and sigh in delight.

> During spring and summer, the yang is abundant externally yet deficient internally; during autumn and winter, the yin is abundant externally yet deficient internally. Yang Jun-Ju has stated, "Above, when it says autumn and winter, this is the time when the yin governs gathering and storage. Here it is restating that during autumn and winter the yin is abundant externally. As for the way of yin and yang, can there be two?" He also stated, "Heaven is yang and earth in yin. Heaven embraces what is outside earth and earth is placed in the midst of heaven.

Both the qi of yin and that of yang emerge from earth and also gather and store in earth. Therefore, it states that which has not yet emerged from earth is known as the yin in the yin; that which has already emerged from the earth is known as the yang in the yin. When it is said that yin governs gathering and storage, it is gathering and storing the yang-qi that has emerged."

With repeated savoring of Zhang Zhi-Cong's marvelous annotation, I came to realize that in spring and summer human yang-qi is drained off externally, and so the internal yang is correspondently exhausted and deficient. Ordinary people need to pay attention and take care to nourish their yang-qi; those who are constitutionally yang deficient should warm and tonify the yang-qi at this time. During autumn and winter, the yang-qi of people is gathered and stored internally, so the yin-essence is correspondently exhausted and deficient. Ordinary people need to pay attention and take care to nourish their yin-essence; those who are constitutionally yin deficient should enrich and tonify their yin-essence at this time. This is nothing more than just going along with the flow of nature. When the famous Song figure Ou-Yang Xiu wrote, "Use the way of nature to nourish a natural body," he was referring to this.

Herb Index

Formula Index

General Index

deficiency-cold patterns, 60
detailed questioning, 89
  value in cough, 90
dialectical materialism, 29
diaphragm disorder, as knotting of three
  yang, 122
diarrhea, 135
  association with dampness, 83
  intestinal rumbling and, 114
  long-term yin depletion from, 83, 86
diazepam, 137
dietary therapy
  for food accumulation cough, 91
  misconceptions about seasonal, 158
different diseases treated similarly, 53, 57
differential diagnosis
  versus biomedical diagnosis, 102
  in canker sores, 124–125
  in chronic pharyngitis, 112
  in diplopia, 146
  in irregular uterine bleeding, 43
  in nasal congestion, 134
  in pediatric coughing and wheezing, 99
  in pediatric diarrhea, 84
  in pediatric high fever, 66
  in pediatric night sweats, 72
  in pediatric nighttime cough, 92
  in pediatric whooping cough, 104
  in pharyngeal pain, 120
  in recurrent hemoptysis, 4
  in recurrent urethral bleeding, 12
  in severe phlegm, 16
  in vaginal discharge, 35
diplopia, 144–150
"Discussion of Blockage of the Nine Orifices
  from Deficiency of the Spleen and Stomach,"
  133
Discussion of Blood Patterns (Xuè zhèng lùn), 15
Discussion of Blood Patterns (Xuè zhèng lùn), 94
Discussion of Cold Damage, 122
Discussion of Cold Damage (Sháng hán lùn), 128
Discussion of Cold Damage (Shāng hán lùn), 24,
  25, 36, 59, 62, 90, 91, 98, 101, 121
    fundamental formula patterns in, 100
Discussion of Cold Damage (Shāng hán lùn),
  26–27, 61
Discussion of Cold Damage (Shāng hán lùn),
  92, 96
*Discussion of Spleen and Stomach Damage
  (Pí wèi lùn)*, 133
disease duration, Bupleurum formulas and, 25
disease location, 139
  defining, 138

disease name
  chronic pharyngitis, 112
  common cold, 66
  deficiency-cold pharyngitis, 120
  food accumulation cough, 92
  food aversion, 78
  hemoptysis, 4
  irregular uterine bleeding, 43
  nasal blockage, 134
  paroxysmal cough, 104
  pediatric coughing and wheezing, 99
  pediatric diarrhea, 84
  pediatric night sweats, 72
  pneumonia with coughing and wheezing, 16
  urethral bleeding, 12
  vaginal discharge, 35
  vision pulled to one side by wind, 146
  whooping cough, 104
disease nature, 139
  in visual distortion, 138
disease stages, 9–10
dispersion disorder, knotting of two yang as,
  122
distending breast pain, 46, 49
*Divine Husbandsman's Classic of the Materia
  Medica (Shén Nóng běn cǎo jīng)*, 17, 36, 44, 53
Divine Pivot (Líng shū), 50, 83, 113, 121, 135,
  141, 146, 152
dizziness, 114, 140, 144
dry stool, in canker sores, 124
dry stools
  in chronic pharyngitis, 110
  in pediatric nighttime cough, 93
  in Spleen yin deficiency, 83
dryness, herbs exacerbating, 17

E

earth
  not generating metal, 95
  nurturing to engender metal, 121
Earth organ disorders, 111
EENT disorders, 109
  chronic pharyngitis, 109–116
  diplopia, 144–150
  nasal congestion, 131–137
  painful throat obstruction, 109–116
  visual distortion, 137–144
effective formulas, caution about changing, 84
*Effective Formulas from Generations of
  Physicians (Shì yī dé xiào fāng)*, 145
eight extraordinary vessels, 50
eighteen incompatibilities (十八反
  shí bā fǎn), 52, 53

M

Translators

Dan Bensky is a graduate of the Macau Institute of Chinese Medicine (Oriental Medicine Diploma, 1975), University of Michigan (B.A. in Chinese Language and Literature, 1978), Michigan State University College of Osteopathic Medicine (Doctor of Osteopathy, 1982), University of Washington (M.A. in Classical Chinese, 1996), and Chinese Academy of Traditional Chinese Medical Sciences (Ph.D. in *Discussion of Cold Damage*, 2006). He contributed to the translation and editing of numerous books, including *Chinese Herbal Medicine: Materia Medica* and *Formulas & Strategies*. A founder of the Seattle Institute of Oriental Medicine, he was awarded in 2008 a Wang Dingyi Cup International Prize for contributions to Chinese medicine.

Andrew Ellis first studied Chinese medicine with Dr. James Tin Yau So at the New England School of Acupuncture. He left New England in 1983 to study Chinese language in Taiwan where he apprenticed with Chinese herbalist Xu Fu-Su for several years. Later he studied internal medicine and gynecology at the Xiamen Hospital of Chinese Medicine. While there, he also specialized in the study of acupuncture with Dr. Shi Neng-Yun and dermatology with Dr. Zhang Guang-Cai. Andrew is the founding owner of Spring Wind Herbs in Berkeley, California and has authored, translated, or co-translated several books on Chinese medicine including *Grasping the Wind*, *The Clinical Experience of Dr. Shi Neng-Yun*, *Notes from South Mountain*, *Fundamentals of Chinese Medicine*, *Chinese Herbal Medicine: Formulas & Strategies*, and *Handbook of Formulas in Chinese Medicine*.

Craig Mitchell, M.S., PH.D., EAMP, is a graduate of the American College of Traditional Chinese Medicine in San Francisco. He studied Chinese language and medicine in Taiwan for several years, and has written numerous articles and translated several

Chinese medical texts including the *Shang Han Lun (On Cold Damage)*. He completed his doctoral degree at the China Academy of Chinese Medical Sciences in 2006. He is now President of the Seattle Institute of Oriental Medicine, where he sees patients, supervises in the clinic, and teaches classes on Chinese herbal medicine and medical Chinese. Craig also maintains a private practice in Seattle.

Michael FitzGerald is a graduate of the bilingual program in Traditional Chinese Medicine at the American College of Traditional Chinese Medicine in San Francisco. He spent several years in Taiwan and Beijing furthering his studies, with a focus on fertility, gastroenterology, cardiac illnesses, and dermatology. He is owner of Stone Mountain Medicine Acupuncture and Herbal Pharmacy in Berkeley, California.